Cancer
The Power of Food
Food, Facts & Recipes

Dr Clare Shaw Recipes by Sara Lewis

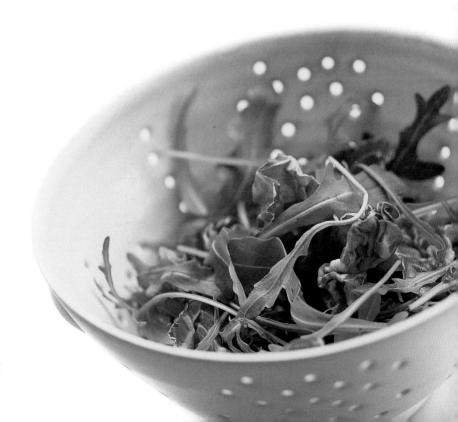

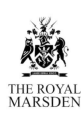

THE ROYAL
MARSDEN

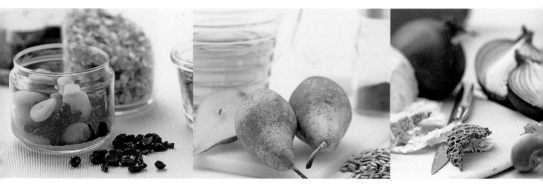

First published in Great Britain in 2005 by
Hamlyn, a division of Octopus Publishing Group Ltd
2–4 Heron Quays, London E14 4JP

ISBN 0 600 61110 8
EAN 9780600611103

A CIP catalogue record for this book is
available from the British Library

Printed and bound in China

10 9 8 7 6 5 4 3 2 1

Nutritional analyses are given per serving.
Where a recipe has split servings (e.g. 'serves
6–8'), the analysis is given for the first figure.

People with known nut allergies should avoid
recipes containing nuts or nut derivatives
and vulnerable people should avoid dishes
containing raw or lightly cooked eggs.

contents

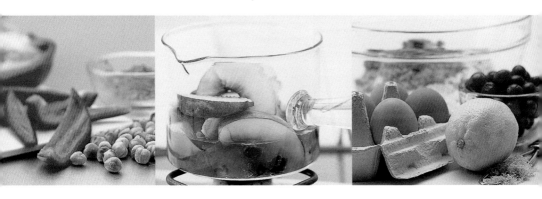

introduction

We all know that the food we eat can influence our health in many ways. Now, evidence would seem to confirm that what we eat affects our chances of developing cancer.

Cancer is a disease that still strikes fear into hearts and minds. Yet, with advances in diagnosis and treatment, many more people are surviving and fewer people now die of cancer than of heart disease in Western countries such as England and the United States of America. In recent years scientists have been turning their attention to how cancer develops and what can cause it. They have identified certain factors in our lifestyles that, although they don't all actually cause cancer, can increase or decrease our risk of developing it.

The story of cancer and how our diet relates to it is as fascinating as it is complex. This book explains concisely how and why our bodies' cells become cancerous and looks at which foods to avoid and which may protect us and reduce the risk of cancer. Following the dietary advice will give a healthy diet with a high intake of vitamins, minerals and other bioactive compounds, and the recipes have been specially formulated to enable you to follow these guidelines. They range from rich smoothies packed full of antioxidants to inspired main dishes drawn from all over the world and delicious bakes and desserts.

The cause of any cancer is seldom straightforward or attributable to a single factor, and it would be naive and wrong to say 'eat X, the magic ingredient, and you won't get cancer.' But diet has been identified as possibly contributing to the risk of a third of all cancers, so eating the right foods can be a great step forward and means that reducing the chance of developing cancer is now a real possibility for us all.

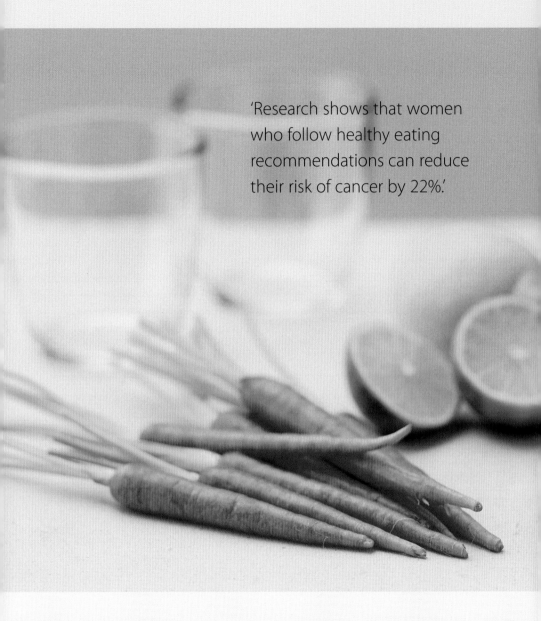

'Research shows that women who follow healthy eating recommendations can reduce their risk of cancer by 22%.'

The recommendations in this book are aimed at healthy people who want to reduce their risk of developing cancer. They do not apply to people who have cancer, and unfortunately there is little research to show us the ideal diet to prevent cancer recurring or new cancers developing.

If you have undergone treatment for cancer, discuss with your doctor whether this diet is suitable for you. Cancer treatment, whether it be surgery, radiotherapy, chemotherapy or some of the new experimental treatments, can leave you with no appetite. In these circumstances there is a risk that you may become malnourished. It is important during treatment that you avoid losing weight, and the diet recommended in this book may not be suitable if you have lost weight unintentionally and do not feel like eating a normal diet. If, however, you have successfully completed anti-cancer treatment, have a good appetite and are able to eat a normal diet, then the recommendations suggested here may be suitable for you.

what is cancer?

Every part of our body is formed of cells that group together to make up our component parts, from our blood and skin to muscles and organs. Cells do not last forever and regularly replace themselves by dividing and multiplying. If any cells lose control over the normal process and begin to multiply out of control they may form a lump or tumour.

Cell replication

A cell's information system, which tells it not only what type of tissue or organ it needs to be but also when and how to replicate itself, is held in the DNA and in the genes in its centre, or nucleus. If this system breaks down or is disrupted, one of three things can happen:

☐ Cells can repair the damage before they multiply.

☐ Cells can die (cells are programmed to die if the DNA is damaged beyond repair).

☐ If neither of these things happens, any damage or mutation to the DNA and protein has the potential to be passed on to new cells, forming a group of abnormal cells. This may be the beginning of a cancer.

'Abnormal cells in the body are not uncommon – the cells usually die before they can continue to multiply.

Not all tumours are cancerous. A non-cancerous growth, called a benign tumour, may be slower to develop and is less likely to cause problems unless it grows very large and perhaps presses on organs within the body. Once benign tumours have been removed they often do not grow back. A tumour made up of cancer cells is what is known as malignant. These tumours are dangerous because they can grow very quickly and can spread around the body.

Because cancer can occur anywhere in the body there are many different types, manifesting a vast range of symptoms, and each can require its own specific treatments.

How cancer spreads

The part of the body in which a tumour first develops is called the primary site, but, in multiplying, cancer cells may invade nearby tissues and organs, affecting the way these function. They can also spread to other tissues or sites; these are called secondary tumours or metastases. Where the cancer cells end up may depend on the position of the primary cancer.

Cancer cells may spread in the bloodstream or in the lymphatic system, which, like the blood circulation system, has a network of tubes throughout the body that collects substances from tissues and circulates them round the body.

When cancer develops in cells of tissues, such as bone marrow, the cancerous cells may be released directly into the bloodstream rather than forming a distinct lump. This type of cancer is called systemic, and it may travel quickly.

'As research progresses, more people then ever before survive cancer.'

what causes cancer?

In addition to basic factors such as age and gender, your chance of developing cancer depends on a balance of a number of elements, and these vary according to the type of cancer.

Environment

Certain compounds – known as carcinogens – can actually cause cancer. The best known is tobacco smoke. Others include the sun, radiation, asbestos and chewing tobacco. Environmental factors mean that the most common types of cancer vary enormously in different parts of the world. One of these factors is diet: what we eat can be either damaging or protective.

Genes

Some cancers, such as colon and breast cancer, may run in families. This does not mean that all members of these families will develop cancer, but they are at higher *risk* than the general population. Much work is being done in this area, and for breast cancer the particular genes that are related to this increased risk have been identified (they are called BRCA1 and BRCA2). But, to keep this in perspective, cancers caused by these genes account for less than 5 per cent of all breast cancers.

'Cancer occurs more often in older people, but there are certain environmental factors that can contribute to its development.'

Viral infections

Some viruses may produce an alteration in the genetic material of cells so they become more susceptible to developing cancer in the future. These infections, which tend to contribute to cancers more in the developing world, include the genital wart virus HPV (cancer of the cervix), hepatitis B (liver cancer) and, in China, Epstein-Barr virus (naso-pharyngeal cancer – that is, of the area behind the nose). Cancer is also seen to occur more frequently in people who have a problem with their immune system, such as those who are taking drugs that suppress the immune system or those who have Aids.

Incidence of cancer

Some types of cancer are a lot more common than others. A record of the numbers of people diagnosed with a new cancer each year and what type of cancer they have is referred to as the incidence rate. It tracks which types of cancer are increasing or decreasing, which are common and which are rare. Although we frequently hear of children and young people with cancer, statistically it is older people who are more likely to get cancer. More and more people are diagnosed with cancer but have successful treatment and are therefore living with the disease.

CANCERS COMMON IN DEVELOPED COUNTRIES
(in descending order of incidence)

Breast

Lung

Large bowel (i.e., colon and rectum)

Prostate

Bladder

Stomach

Non-Hodgkin's lymphoma

Head and neck cancer

Oesophagus

Pancreas

Malignant melanoma

Leukaemia

Ovary

Kidney

Uterus

Brain

Myeloma

Cervix

diet and cancer

There is a lot of contradictory information available about diet and cancer, so it is important to understand a little of how studies are carried out to help you to make up your own mind about various claims.

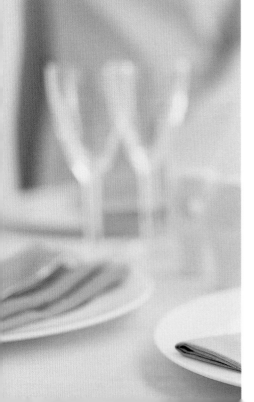

'It is thought that approximately one-third of all cancers may be linked to diet.'

What research tells us

Many of the early theories on the links between diet and cancer were tested in the laboratory and on animals. These provided helpful leads, but chemicals often react in quite different ways in humans than they do on animals or in a test tube. Also, it is not safe to assume that links found in animals equally apply to humans. The best information comes from studying human beings.

Types of study

Epidemiological studies look at what people eat alongside the incidence of cancer, and because dietary habits vary enormously these can produce a wealth of information on how diet may affect health.

Migrant studies provide useful information on dietary and genetic factors. When Japanese people migrated to Hawaii, for example, their dietary patterns changed – and so did their risk of certain cancers. As the traditional Japanese diet has become more Westernized so rates of breast and colon cancer have increased. These studies also illustrate that environment, rather than just individual genetic make-up, is a factor.

Case control studies investigate the links that can be deduced by comparing diets of cancer patients with similar people who do not have cancer. These tend to yield the best results when there is a big difference between the diets of those with and without cancer.

Cohort studies follow the health and diet of healthy people over a long period of time to see if there is any difference in the diets of those who develop cancer and those who don't.

Intervention studies track results from a particular diet or supplement, using a control group that is not given the diet or supplement. Ethically, of course, people should not be exposed to substances thought to increase the risk of cancer, so these studies are on particular nutrients thought to protect against cancer. 'Double blind' trials – when neither the researchers nor the individuals know which group they belong to – produce the most reliable results.

Some research may indicate a link between diet and cancer, while other research may provide more conclusive results. Where evidence is sufficiently strong, prestigious organizations such as the World Cancer Research Fund and the World Health Organization publish guidance to help people make dietary changes.

SORTING THE WHEAT FROM THE CHAFF

Validity of research results can depend on factors such as:

How the studies have been conducted – on humans, animals or on cells in a laboratory

Rigour of testing – Were the people in the study alike in many of their characteristics, or could they bring too many other variables into the equation?

Reliability of record – Have the figures depended, for example, on people's recollection of what they consumed a long time ago?

dietary influences

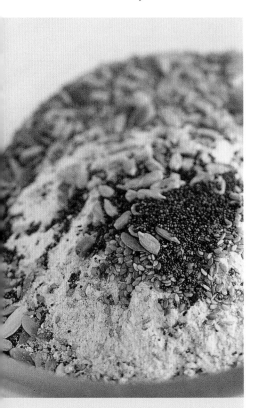

Studies over many years have shown a number of interesting correlations between different diets and cancers.

- ☐ The incidence of certain cancers, especially stomach and bowel, has increased as large-scale food processing has replaced many of the wholegrain cereals, pulses and roots in our diet with white flour and refined cereals and sugars.

- ☐ Cancers of the stomach and oesophagus are much less common where the typical diet is high in cereals, tubers and starchy foods – often providing half of the dietary energy needs – but low in animal proteins (meat and dairy products). Diets in developed countries tend to be high in animal proteins, sugar and salt, but low in starches.

- ☐ There is a greater incidence of stomach cancer in countries where traditionally a lot of salty foods are eaten – for example, Japan, China and Portugal.

- ☐ In southern European countries, the consumption of fruit and vegetables is generally higher than in northern Europe, and the incidence of cancers of the mouth and throat, oesophagus, lung and stomach is lower in the south.

'Large-scale food processing has replaced many of the wholegrain cereals, pulses and roots in our diet.'

How can diet influence the development of cancer?

A damaged cell needs to replicate in order to grow into a group of cancer cells (see page 6). Some substances in our diet may either encourage the replication process and promote cancer growth or slow it down, so protecting against cancer.

Carcinogenic agents

These agents may directly influence DNA or protein in cells. Examples include aflatoxins, which are found in mouldy food (see page 26), alcohol (see page 25) and certain compounds produced by some cooking and food-processing methods (see page 26).

Tumour promoters

Unlike carcinogens, tumour promoters do not act directly on DNA, but they stimulate the genes and encourage replication. Some hormones may act in this way, and although the body produces these hormones naturally, diet can affect the level of, for example, oestrogens in the body (see page 22). Other tumour promoters include alcohol and a high-fat or high-energy diet, which may promote the production of harmful substances, such as free radicals. Free radicals are thought to influence DNA disorganization.

But, just as we may introduce harmful elements into our bodies through our diet, there are also nutrients that may protect us.

'Cancers of the stomach and oesophagus are much less common where the typical diet is high in cereals, tubers and starchy foods.'

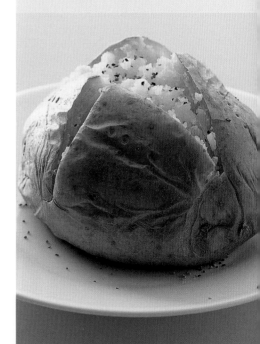

protective nutrients

Many foods contain protective substances that may reduce damage to tissues by free radicals (see page 13) or potentially reduce cell growth.

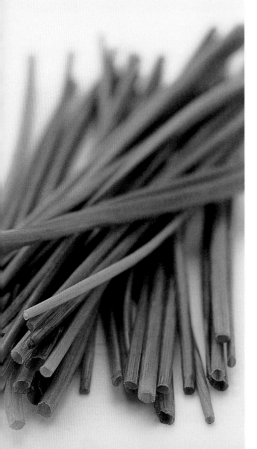

'Certain nutrients may slow down or delay the progress of tumour growth.'

Antioxidants

Antioxidants are important constituents of the diet and are involved in DNA and cell maintenance and repair. They may reduce the production of free radicals, preventing early damage to cells and so reducing the chance that they will become cancerous. Antioxidants in the diet may be in the form of vitamins or minerals, such as vitamins C and E, beta-carotene and selenium, or they may be found in flavonoids in vegetables (see opposite).

Phytoestrogens

Phytoestrogens have properties similar to oestrogens, but they are much weaker than the oestrogens the body itself produces. They can be divided primarily into two groups: isoflavones and lignans. Isoflavones are linked to the protein part of food and lignans to the fibre. The table opposite includes examples of sources of phytoestrogens.

Other bioactive compounds

Many foods have functions beyond the vitamins and minerals they contain. Research is revealing that some of their chemicals and reactions may be beneficial to health. In laboratory experiments, for example, garlic extracts have killed *Heliobacter pylori*, a bacteria that can grow in the stomach and is known to increase the risk of cancer. Sulphur-containing compounds in garlic and onions may also reduce the formation of carcinogenic compounds that arise from the curing of meats (see page 20).

VITAMINS AND MINERALS	POSITIVE FUNCTION	SOURCES
Carotenoids These are precursors of vitamin A; they include alpha-carotene, beta-carotene, xanthophylls (the main one is lutein), lycopene, cryptoxanthin	Antioxidant	Dark green leafy vegetables, orange vegetables and fruit. LUTEIN: kale, spinach, broccoli, corn LYCOPENE: tomatoes, watermelons, pink grapefruit, guavas CRYPTOXANTHIN: mangoes, papayas, persimmons, red peppers, pumpkins
Folate (folic acid)	Antioxidant; may affect division of cells in the colon	Beans, green leafy vegetables, liver, nuts, wholegrain cereals
Selenium	Stimulation of detoxification enzymes	Brazil nuts, bread, eggs, fish, meat
Vitamin C (ascorbic acid)	Antioxidant	Broccoli, cabbage and other green leafy vegetables, citrus fruit, mangoes, peppers, strawberries, tomatoes
Vitamin D	May control cell growth through its effect on calcium	Sunlight
Vitamin E	Antioxidant	Nuts, seeds, vegetable oils, wheatgerm, wholegrains

OTHER BIOACTIVE COMPOUNDS	POSITIVE FUNCTION	SOURCES
Allium compounds (contain sulphur)	Stimulate detoxification enzymes	Chives, garlic, onions
Flavonoids (e.g. quercetin)	Antioxidant function within the plant	Berries, broad beans, broccoli, onions, tomatoes
Isothiocyanates	Stimulate detoxifying enzymes	Broccoli, Brussels sprouts, cabbage and other brassicas
Phytoestrogens (isoflavones and lignans)	May alter steroid hormone metabolism	ISOFLAVONES: beans, chickpeas, lentils, soya LIGNANS: oil seeds (e.g. flax, soya, rape), legumes and various other vegetables and fruit, particularly berries, wholegrains
Plant sterols	May bind with hormones in the gut and influence hormone metabolism	Cereals, fruit, nuts, seeds, vegetables
Terpenoid (e.g. D-limonene)	Stimulate enzyme systems	Oil of lemons, oranges and other citrus fruits

starchy and protein-rich foods

Starchy foods include cereals, such as wheat, rye, oats, barley and rice, and some vegetables, such as potatoes, sweet potatoes and yams. These foods should be the basis of your diet.

SINGLE PORTION GUIDANCE

Cereals, pasta and noodles

2 tablespoons cooked rice
(medium serving = 2 portions)

80 g (3¼ oz) cooked pasta or noodles
(average serving = 3 portions)

small portion cooked porridge
(average serving = 2 portions)

5 tablespoons muesli

2 tablespoons cooked barley

Bread

2 medium slices wholemeal bread

1 wholemeal muffin

2 small wholemeal rolls

3 slices rye bread

2 bagels

½ naan bread

1 large chapatti

1 small pitta bread

Pulses

3 tablespoons cooked lentils or pulses,
such as red kidney, haricot and
borlotti beans or split peas

2–3 tablespoons cooked chickpeas

3 level tablespoons hummus

Others

½ medium jacket potato

1 medium sweet potato

1 medium banana

½ plantain (NB: plantains should
always be eaten cooked)

Food starch and plant proteins are high in a number of nutrients that may protect against cancer:

- ☐ fibre (non-starch polysaccharides or NSP)
- ☐ vitamins (particularly B vitamins)
- ☐ carotenoids (in sweet potatoes and yams)
- ☐ folate (in pulses)
- ☐ vitamin E (in wholegrain cereals)
- ☐ vitamin C (in potatoes and pulses but see also page 18).

Many researchers considered initially that fibre was the most important constituent of wholegrain cereals, but it appears that this may instead be the combination of all nutrients. It seems that eating refined cereal foods is not protective against cancer, so choose grains that have not had the husk and germ removed through processing.

In areas of the world where people eat a diet high in wholegrain cereals, pulses, legumes, roots and tubers, less meat, fat, sugar and salt are often eaten. This balance appears to help reduce the rate of cancer of the stomach, colon and rectum. This sort of diet is also lower in energy, so it is a good way to control body weight (see page 28). A monotonous diet that does not include vegetables increases the risk of cancer of the oesophagus.

Get protein from plants as an alternative to meat and fish. Eat more pulses, such as beans and lentils, and try nuts and seeds for extra flavour, texture and variety.

Getting the most from starch and plant proteins

Aim to eat 600–800 g (1¼–1¾ lb) or seven portions of starchy and protein-rich plant foods each day (see opposite). It is important to have variety in such a starchy diet to ensure a wide range of vitamins and minerals – a huge bowl of brown rice twice a day is not the answer! These foods are bulky and make you feel full, so you should naturally reduce your intake of fat, meat and sugar, altering the balance of each meal.

+ Add pulses to casseroles and stews.

+ Use oatmeal and oat flakes to add texture to homemade bread or to top crumbles.

+ Whenever possible, choose wholegrain cereals, such as brown rice and wholemeal bread, rather than white.

+ A bowl of muesli with a chopped banana will provide two portions to begin the day.

+ Add a handful of chopped nuts, such as walnuts, to stir-fries.

+ Sprinkle toasted sesame or pumpkin seeds over salads.

Simple ways to include more of these foods …

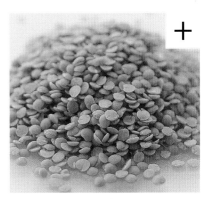

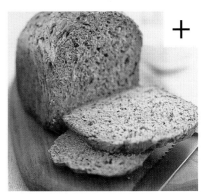

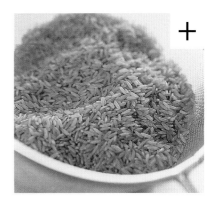

vegetables and fruit

Diets high in vegetables and fruit tend to be rich in the vitamins, minerals and compounds that help protect against cancer (see pages 14–15), in particular cancers of the mouth and pharynx, oesophagus, lung, stomach, colon and rectum, and also possibly the pancreas, breast and bladder. It is difficult to assess how much of these substances the body requires to help protect against diseases, but by choosing a wide variety of vegetables and fruit the chances of eating more of these substances is increased.

SINGLE PORTION GUIDANCE

1 medium apple

3 dried apricots

5 tablespoons beansprouts

2 spears broccoli

3 heaped tablespoons cabbage, shredded

3 heaped tablespoons sliced carrots

5 cm (2 in) piece cucumber

1 heaped tablespoon dried fruit

3 heaped tablespoons fruit salad

½ grapefruit

1 orange or 2 tangerines, satsumas etc.

3 heaped tablespoons peas/green beans

½ fresh pepper

green side salad

What and how much?

To get the full benefit from your diet you should aim for five or more portions a day – this should add up to around 400–800 g (13 oz–1¾ lb) of vegetables and fruit every day, all year round. Include vegetables and fruit in season to make the most of the best vitamin and mineral content and to add variety to your diet.

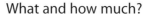

□ Starchy vegetables, such as potatoes, sweet potatoes and yams can be important contributors to your diet (see page 16) but should not be counted in your five fruit/ vegetables portions a day.

□ Pulses do not contain quite as many vitamins as other vegetables so eat only one portion a day.

□ Count fruit juice as only one portion in the day, because it does not contain fibre.

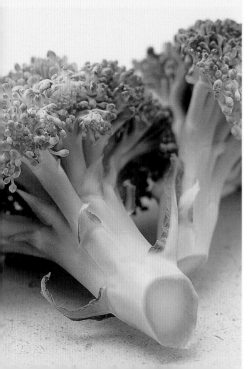

+ A glass of fruit juice first thing in the morning is one portion to start you off for the day. Be alert to juice look-alikes, described as 'juice drinks', 'hi-juice' and the like, because these are not 100 per cent fruit juice.

+ Boost your intake of vegetables by having a vegetarian meal once a week.

+ Whizz up delicious fruit smoothies; unlike plain juice they contain all the fibre of the whole fruit.

+ If you need to nibble between meals, graze on dried fruit – try some of the more unusual ones, such as cranberries and blueberries.

+ Add colour and extra nutrition to leafy salads with slivers of red pepper, raw carrot or beetroot.

Simple ways to include more of these foods...

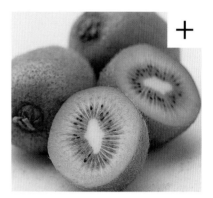

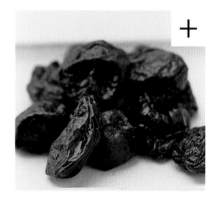

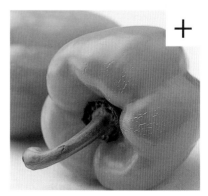

meat, fish and eggs

Meat, fish and eggs provide us with protein, vitamins and minerals, but the typical Western diet relies too heavily on these foods at the expense of starches and vegetables.

PROCESSED MEATS AND FISH

Curing, as in the production of bacon, ham and kippers, uses nitrates and nitrites that preserve the meat or fish against bacteria; they also give processed meats their characteristic pink colour. In the stomach the nitrites may be converted into nitrosamines, suspected of being cancer producing.

Smoking meat or fish produces polycyclic aromatic hydrocarbons from the burning wood. Studies on humans have failed to show categorically that these increase the risk of cancer but animal experiments have raised concerns. Smoked food is often also salted and may represent additional risk for cancer of the stomach.

Eat cured or smoked meat only occasionally.

Red meat

High consumption of red meat may increase chances of colorectal cancer and possibly cancers of the pancreas, breast, prostate and kidney. It is unclear exactly how eating a lot of meat and processed meats increases the risk of colorectal cancer, but it may be due in part to an association with a high fat intake. Limit your red meat intake to less than 80 g (3¼ oz) daily, or if you eat larger portions, redress the balance with meat-free days.

Poultry

Poultry does not appear to be linked to an increased risk of any type of cancer, so this would be a good alternative to red meat.

Fish

Fish may help protect against cancers of the colon, rectum, breast and ovary. However, it is not known if this is due to fish alone or to the effect of replacing meat in the diet. Experimental work on breast cancer has suggested that omega-3 fatty acids in oily fish may reduce the growth of cancer cells in animals. There is not enough evidence to be able to recommend fish oils specifically as a protective ingredient against breast cancer, but they are a general asset in the diet.

Eggs

Any association of eggs with an increase in risk of cancer is considered very weak, so they can be a useful alternative to meat as a source of protein.

+ If you eat red meat, choose lean red meat rather than processed meat products.

+ Oily fish, such as salmon and sardines, is a healthy choice and quick and easy to cook.

+ Try meat from non-domesticated or free-range animals, such as deer or rabbit.

+ White fish is very low in fat; jazz it up with a Mediterranean-style crust (see page 82).

+ Chicken is one of the most adaptable meats; choose a free-range bird for maximum flavour.

Simple ways to include more of these foods…

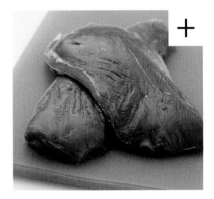

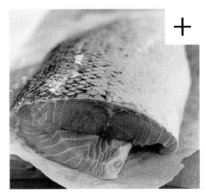

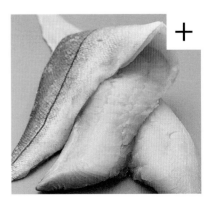

fats and oils

Some, but not all, reports suggest that a high-fat diet may increase the possibility of cancers of the colon, rectum, breast, prostate and lung.

DO WE NEED FATS AT ALL?

Our bodies are unable to make some essential fatty acids, and we get these from vegetable seed oils. The body requires only small amounts, and they are easily consumed within a low-fat diet. (These essential fats are not present in vegetable oil that has been completely hydrogenated, although many soft margarines do contain such fatty acids.)

Dairy products are largely saturated fat, which is also a good source of calcium, necessary for bone formation, and the oils in oily fish are beneficial in a diet in general, although they have no proven protective role against cancer.

Cutting down on fats, especially saturated fats, is sensible advice for health in general, but as direct protection against cancer this is, perhaps, the weakest when it comes to good evidence. Much work has been done on whether fat in the diet increases the risk of breast cancer, but the available evidence is not strong. Studies measuring female hormones, oestrogens, have failed to show changes in levels when women eat a high-fat diet, so it is likely that fat may act via its influence on obesity (see page 28).

Ways to cut down on fat:
- Avoid too much fatty food, particularly of animal origin, and have fewer creamy desserts and rich creamy sauces.
- Avoid snacks high in fat such as crisps, deep-fried snacks, salted nuts and chocolate.
- Choose lean cuts of meat and poultry without the skin.
- Use unsaturated fats in place of saturated fats but moderate your intake of all fats.
- Reduce the amount of oil or fat used in cooking and choose monounsaturated fats (e.g. olive oil) when possible.
- Choose low-fat dairy products to provide calcium without excess saturated fat.
- Look for labels on margarines that refer to cis fatty acids; avoid trans fats.

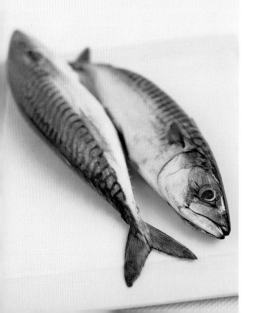

Positive fats

Simple changes to your diet enable you to reduce your fat intake and switch to mono and unsaturated fats.

+ Use chopped nuts or avocado instead of creamy dressings to liven up a green salad.

+ Experiment with an oil/water spray – try it on lean pork steaks, for example, accompanied with steamed vegetables and a jacket potato for a healthy supper.

+ Dip bruschetta into a garlic-infused olive oil rather than using butter.

Simple ways to include more of these foods…

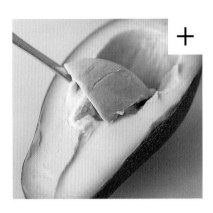

TYPES OF FATS AND OILS	ORIGIN	SOURCE
Saturated	Mostly of animal origin, but also coconut and palm oils; tends to be solid at room temperature	Butter, lard, cheese, fat on meat
Polyunsaturated	Mostly of vegetable origin; tends to be liquid at room temperature	Oily fish, avocados, nuts, rapeseed, safflower, sunflower and corn oils
Monounsaturated	Found in fish and some nuts and seeds	Olive oil; also some other oils and polyunsaturates
Hydrogenated Comes in two forms: trans fats and cis fatty acids (a naturally occurring form that is preferable to trans fats)	Produced by a chemical process that solidifies a liquid oil; the altered chemical structure can affect the way it reacts in the body	Used in processed foods, including margarines, biscuits, cakes, pastry

salt

A lot of salt in your diet increases the risk of stomach cancer. This is seen particularly in countries such as China, Japan and in Hawaii, where foods like salted fish and pickled vegetables are popular.

FOODS HIGH IN SALT INCLUDE:

Ham and bacon

Cheese

Prepared sauces and soups

Crisps

Salted fish and vegetables

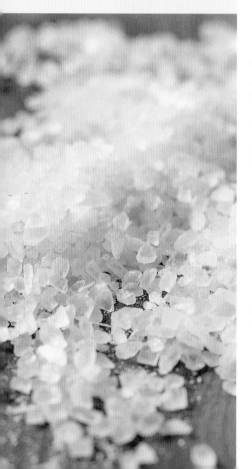

It is probable that the salt is not itself carcinogenic, but it can damage the lining of the stomach. As the cells multiply to try to repair the damage, the extra activity may increase the chances of cancer cells forming. The damage can also leave the stomach lining vulnerable to carcinogens.

Not only do we sprinkle salt on our food and add it as we cook, but manufactured foods, from snacks and pies to bottled sauces, often contain large amounts of 'hidden' salt. Aim to limit your total intake to less than 6 g (¼ oz or about 1¼ teaspoons) a day.

top tips

☐ Check labelling carefully and reduce the amount of processed foods you eat.

☐ Limit your intake of particularly salty foods.

☐ Remember that sea salt contains the same amount of sodium chloride as table salt.

☐ Use herbs and spices, instead of salt, to enhance the flavour of food (there are plenty of ideas in the recipe section).

alcohol

If you like alcohol, then enjoy a unit or two each day with your meal and avoid binge drinking. It is the pattern of drinking and the amount you consume that are important factors. Less concentrated drinks such as beer and wine are better choices than spirits.

Alcoholic drinks increase the risk of a number of cancers, notably mouth, pharynx and larynx, oesophagus and liver. People who develop alcoholic cirrhosis also have a higher risk of liver cancer. Alcohol has been shown to increase the risk of breast cancer, with the risk becoming greater as the amount drunk on a daily basis increases. The way in which this works is not known, but it may be by its action on hormone levels. Alcohol may also increase the risk of colon and rectum cancer and is associated with other problems, such as heart disease and stroke.

The action of alcohol is intensified if you smoke, particularly with respect to cancers of the mouth and throat.

HOW MUCH IS 'ONE DRINK'?

1 small glass (125 ml/4 fl oz) 8% wine
= 1 drink

1 glass (140 ml/5 fl oz) 10% champagne
= 1½ drinks

1 large glass (175 ml/6 fl oz) 12% red wine
= 2 drinks

600 ml (1 pint) 3% draught beer
= 1½ drinks

600 ml (1 pint) 5% beer or lager
= 3 drinks

600 ml (1 pint) strong (6%) beer
= 3½ drinks

600 ml (1 pint) dry cider = 2 drinks

60 ml (2 fl oz) sherry = 1 drink

30 ml (1 fl oz) spirits = 1 drink

top tips
- ☐ Limit your daily alcohol to fewer than two drinks for men and one for women.
- ☐ Check the alcoholic content of drinks, including wine – a 150 ml (5 fl oz) glass of wine with 13% alcohol equates to two drinks.
- ☐ Broaden your choice of non-alcoholic drinks: try delicious fruit juices and smoothies.
- ☐ Have an alcohol-free day each week.

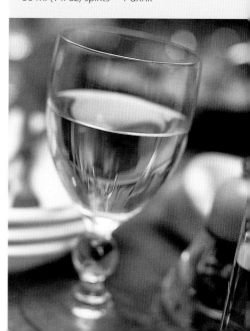

maximum goodness

How fresh food is and the way it is cooked make a huge difference to its nutritional value and therefore to its effectiveness in protecting against cancer

Freshness

The vitamin and mineral content of vegetables and fruit begin to deteriorate as soon as they are picked, and exposure to light, heat and damp can further reduce the nutritional value.

As it ages, food, especially when stored poorly, can be a source of bacteria or fungal contamination. Liver cancer, for example, has been associated with eating food contaminated with aflatoxins produced by the fungus *Aspergillus flavus* and *Aspergillus parasiticus* found to grow on peanuts. Contamination begins before it is visible, so apparently 'clean' food may already contain toxicants.

Cooking meat and fish

Cooking meat and fish at very high temperatures, and particularly over an open flame, is likely to produce heterocyclic aromatic amines. These are known carcinogens in animals, and there is concern that they act in a similar way on humans, so it is advisable to eat food that has been barbecued only in moderation, and where possible to avoid charred meat and meat juices altogether.

Vegetables and fruit

Heat destroys some nutrients, and some are also lost by leaching out into water, so cook vegetables and fruit for as short a time as possible, and steam or bake rather than boil them to preserve their vitamin and mineral content.

'Fresh foods tend to have a vitamin and mineral content that are beneficial for good health.'

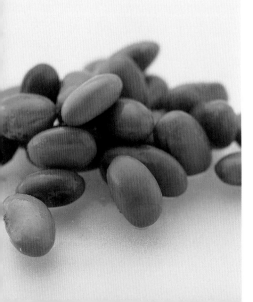

Avoid preparing vegetables too far in advance, because vitamins are lost from the cut surface that is exposed to the air.

Eating fruit and vegetables raw will enable you to benefit from the least loss of nutrients, and many are enjoyable this way, but there are exceptions. Some foods, notably red kidney beans, contain natural toxins that need to be destroyed by cooking at sufficiently high temperatures.

top tips

- ☐ Only buy food that looks fresh and is within its best-before date.
- ☐ Avoid damaged fruit and vegetables as these will attract mould more easily.
- ☐ Look for locally grown food and food in season; less time is likely to have passed since harvesting.
- ☐ Store fruit and vegetables in a cool, dark place and check them regularly – discarding any that develop bruises or that become discoloured.
- ☐ Store cooked and raw meats separately; any bacteria in raw meat should be killed by cooking but could migrate to the cooked food and multiply.
- ☐ If a food shows any sign of mould, throw it all away, don't just cut off the affected part.
- ☐ Throw away food that tastes 'off' or has an unusual bitter taste.

MICROWAVES

Cooking in a microwave can help preserve the nutrients in vegetables and fruit, because it uses minimal water. As with other methods, avoid overcooking, which will destroy some vitamins.

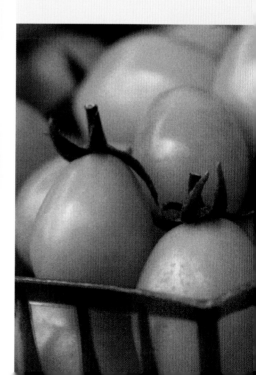

weight and exercise

Obesity may increase the risk of cancer, including cancers of the endometrium, kidney and possibly the colon, in a number of ways. Putting on a lot of weight means an increase in cell replication, so enhancing the chances of cancer cells developing. An overweight person also has more body fat in which to store higher amounts of chemical carcinogens. Increased production of hormones in body fat may also be a factor.

CALCULATING YOUR BODY MASS INDEX (BMI)

Note your weight in kilos

Note your height in metres

Work out the following on a calculator:

weight (kg) ÷ height $(m)^2$

OR

weight (lb) x 700 ÷ height $(in)^2$

The result is your BMI.

18.5–25	normal
over 25	overweight
over 30	obese

If you have any particular concerns about your health or weight, consult your doctor or dietitian.

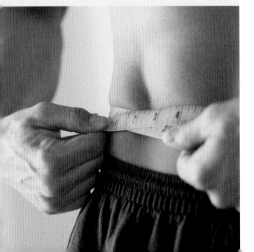

Women, the menopause and breast cancer

Obesity increases the risk of breast cancer in post-menopausal women by about 50 per cent. But why? It may be the effect on the body's hormone levels. After the menopause women continue to produce hormones in fat, so fat women can potentially produce greater amounts. It has been shown, for example, that taller women have an increased risk of post-menopausal breast cancer, perhaps due to increased exposure to hormones throughout their lifetime.

Obesity does not increase breast cancer risk in pre-menopausal women – but a fat pre-menopausal woman is likely to become a fat post-menopausal woman, so being overweight carries the potential for risk in any adult woman .

This hormonal explanation is thought to be similar for women who develop endometrial cancer, although in this instance the links with obesity hold for both pre- and post-menopausal women.

Exercise

Although not strictly a dietary recommendation, physical inactivity and excess weight are linked, and together have been estimated to account for approximately one-fifth to one-third of several of the most common cancers such as those of the breast (post-menopausal), colon and endometrium.

If you regularly take in more energy (in the form of food) than you use, you will put on weight. As people become more sedentary and eat high-energy diets, obesity becomes more common. This is particularly noticeable in Western populations, where obesity has risen dramatically over recent years.

People with active jobs are less likely to have to plan to exercise, but if your typical daily activity level is low, try to walk briskly for an hour each day. Take more vigorous exercise for an hour each week. If you are unsure of how much exercise you can do, always check with your doctor.

top tips

- ☐ Starchy foods, fruit and vegetables are bulky, filling and not high in energy.
- ☐ Cut down on fats (animal and vegetable fats both contain the same amount of energy).
- ☐ If you are overweight, try to make dietary changes for life. This will help you keep your new lower weight.
- ☐ Reduce portion sizes but increase the variety of what you eat.
- ☐ Increase the amount of exercise you do.

'Try to walk briskly for at least an hour every day.'

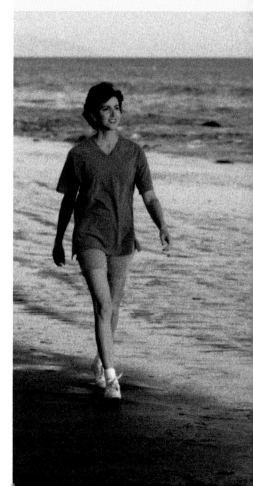

some questions answered

Are fruit and vegetables better raw than cooked?
▶

Because some of the vitamins are destroyed during storage and cooking, raw or very lightly cooked fresh vegetables and fruit are likely to have a higher vitamin content. However, cooking may help make vitamins more available for absorption – the body absorbs beta-carotene better from cooked carrots, for example.

Is a vegetarian/vegan diet a good idea?
▶

Strict vegetarian diets that include only a few basic foods are often not healthy because they may lack the necessary energy, protein, vitamins and minerals. Variety is important. All the international recommendations for the healthiest diet to protect against many different types of cancer do not rule out a modest amount of animal protein but do mean a shift in favour of cereals, fruit and vegetables.

Is organic food healthier?
▶

There is no consistent data to show that organic foods are necessarily more nutritious, although people may choose such foods because they feel they taste better or out of concern for the environment. The nutritional content of the food we eat is dependent on many factors, including growing conditions, the variety of crop or breed, the nutrient content of the soil and storage conditions. As some plant nutrients deteriorate with time after harvesting it is particularly important that food is eaten fresh. This applies to both organically and non-organically produced food.

If I can afford only a small amount of organic food, which should I choose?
▶

It is important to try to choose foods that are fresh, so why not find out if there is a local farmers' market near you. Food that is produced locally is likely to be in season and not be stored for long periods of time.

Are genetically modified foods carcinogenic?

▶

The influence of diet on cancer risk generally takes effect over a long period of time, often many years, and tends to relate to the balance of various foods rather than any particular food being identified as a cause of the cancer. This makes the assessment of genetically modified foods difficult as they have not been monitored for long enough to know whether they can influence risk for better or for worse.

Should I eat soya food

▶

The potential health benefits to be derived from eating soya-based foods has led to an increase in interest in them. They also contain plant-derived compounds known as phytoestrogens (see page 14). Although there appears to be a theoretical reason for their protective effect against hormone cancers, there is currently insufficient evidence that they reduce the risk of breast cancer. However, soya products, such as meat substitutes and non-dairy milks and yogurts are useful both to strict vegetarians and people with an intolerance to milk.

Can't I just take a vitamin pill to boost my intake of antioxidants?

▶

All research identifying vitamins and minerals that may protect against cancer has also discovered that it is the whole food containing these vitamins that is the most important aspect of protection, not the vitamins alone. There are studies that have shown antioxidant vitamin supplements decreasing the risk of certain cancers in poorly nourished individuals, but there appears to be no benefit if you are well nourished. So, exciting though it would be if an antioxidant 'magic bullet' could prevent cancerous cells from growing, it is not as easy as that.

Are tea and coffee good or bad news? ▶

Although some early studies suggested a link between coffee drinking and bladder cancer, later research has failed to substantiate these claims. Very hot drinks are to be avoided, however, because they may cause damage to the oesophagus and increase the risk of cancer. Research into the antioxidant activity of chemicals found in tea and coffee may prove useful in the future.

Is it true that some foods may contain dioxin? ▶

Dioxins are chlorine-containing organic substances. Although they can be produced naturally, they most commonly enter the food chain as by-products of some industrial processes and waste incineration. Dioxins are known to be carcinogenic in humans, and the World Health Organization has set up a global programme to monitor food contamination. This programme identifies maximum doses that should not be exceeded.

Dioxins dissolve in fat. They are therefore stored within the body and can take a number of years to break down. To reduce exposure to dioxins, trim fat from meat and choose low-fat dairy products. Cooking food may reduce its dioxin content, and a balanced diet from a variety of foods will avoid excessive exposure from a single source.

What is a co-carcinogen? ▶

A co-carcinogen is anything that, when combined with a carcinogenic substance, enhances the activity of the carcinogen.

Can food additives cause cancer? ▶

Most manufactured foods contain preservatives, colouring agents, emulsifiers, stabilizers or sweeteners. Those that rigorous testing has shown to be toxic are no longer used or strictly limited. Some have been used over many years without apparent side-effects and are generally recognized as safe, and regulations are thought to be sufficient to make allowance for interactions between different additives. At present dietary studies have not identified any link between additives and the risk of cancer, but tests continue, and using fresh ingredients whenever possible will keep your intake of additives to a minimum.

I thought alcohol was protective against heart disease? ▶

Alcohol has been shown to produce a small increase in the proportion of 'good' HDL (high density lipoprotein) cholesterol in the bloodstream. This effect can be produced by other factors, including exercise. Studies that have shown a possible benefit to the heart of drinking wine have suggested that this is possibly due to the antioxidants in wine, such as flavonoids. It cannot be ruled out, however, that these results may be due to other factors, such as exercise, eating more fruit and vegetables or eating less saturated fat.

Does this mean that it is good to drink alcohol? ▶

Because higher intakes of alcohol contribute to an increase in heart disease, strokes, some cancers and high blood pressure, the advice for heart disease and cancer is the same: if you drink alcohol, drink in moderation.

Apart from changing my diet, is there anything else I can do to reduce the risk of cancer?
▶

Yes, there are a number of things that influence cancer risk apart from diet:

☐ Stop smoking and avoid passive smoking. Smoking is thought to account for 90 per cent of all lung cancers and contribute to a number of other cancers including bladder, kidney, cervix, throat and mouth, oesophagus, pancreas and stomach.

☐ Minimize exposure to ultraviolet light from sunbeds and excessive exposure to sunlight.

☐ Adopt a healthy lifestyle by taking physical activity.

Are pesticides used on food carcinogenic?
▶

Expert committees set safety standards for all approved pesticides, based on scientific evidence. Eating foods containing pesticide residues at levels below the safety limits should not harm people's health. Not eating any fruit and vegetables would be a much bigger risk to your health than eating foods containing low levels of pesticide residues.

I've heard that high-baked foods like crisps and crispbreads contain acrylamide, a highly carcinogenic chemical. Is this true?
▶

Acrylamide is a contaminant from the rubber industry, but it has also been found to form in starch-based foods, such as potato chips, French fries, cereals and bread that have been cooked at high temperatures. In animal experiments it was identified as a possible cause of cancer in humans, but to what extent it actually affects human cancer is not known. Much more research is needed to help answer this question.

Does smoking deprive your body of vitamins? ▶

Smoking reduces the level of vitamins in the bloodstream, particularly vitamin C. So stopping smoking may improve nutrient levels as well as reducing cancer risk.

Will a high-protein, low-carbohydrate weight-reducing diet affect my risk of cancer? ▶

Yes, it might. All the evidence for diet being protective indicates that your diet should contain plenty of starchy foods, fruit and vegetables with small portions of animal protein.

Does eating dairy produce cause cancer? ▶

The evidence is inconclusive – for every study showing an increased risk of cancer there are others suggesting this is not the case. Choose low-fat dairy products that may help reduce the risk of heart disease.

I have a friend who follows a very healthy diet but she still got cancer. ▶

Unfortunately there are no guarantees in life. The recommendations in this book are thought to influence your risk of developing some cancers. Not all cancers are influenced by diet. There are many causes of cancer, known and unknown, so these recommendations are all about trying to reduce risk while having a healthy and delicious diet.

Is this diet suitable for my children? ▶

Whilst this the recipes in this book are suitable for children they may require additional high-energy foods to help them grow. Also particularly important for children are moderate amounts of dairy products, meat, fish or alternatives such as eggs, beans and lentils. This will provide some of the necessary vitamins and minerals such as vitamin D, calcium and iron for growth and development. By including fruit, vegetables and cereal-based foods in the diet you are establishing good healthy eating habits for the future.

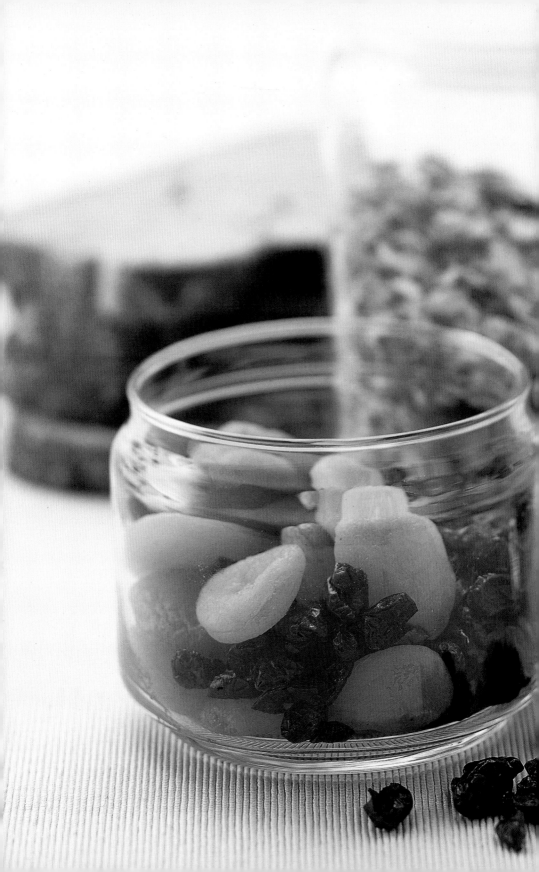

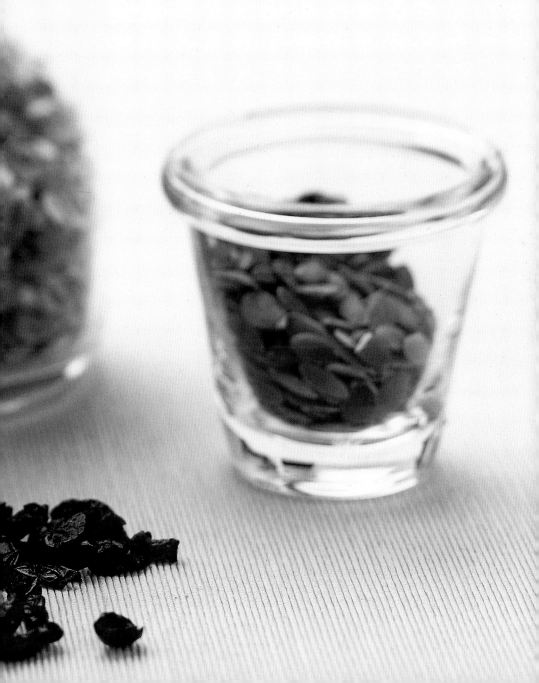

breakfasts

Nutritional values
Kcals 245 (1020 Kj)
fat 13 g
protein 3 g
carbohydrate 30 g
Good source of fibre

Preparation time
20 minutes
Cooking time
30–35 minutes
Makes
10

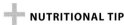 **NUTRITIONAL TIP**
Start your day with this delicious high-fibre bar that also provides iron, zinc and magnesium.

double-decker muesli bars

These moist oaty bars have a naturally sweet ribbon of prunes running through the centre. Make them at the weekend and keep them in the biscuit tin for those weekday mornings when you need breakfast in a hurry.

150 g (5 oz) vegetable margarine or butter

75 g (3 oz) light muscovado sugar

2 tablespoons golden syrup

75 g (3 oz) wholemeal plain flour

200 g (7 oz) muesli, plus 3 tablespoons for sprinkling

3 tablespoons wheatgerm

200 g (7 oz) ready-to-eat dried prunes, finely chopped

1 Line a shallow 20 cm (8 inch) square cake tin with a large piece of nonstick baking paper, snipping into the corners so that it fits the base and sides of the tin snugly.

2 Put the margarine or butter, sugar and syrup in a saucepan and heat gently until the fat has melted and the sugar has dissolved.

3 Take the pan off the heat and stir in the flour, muesli and wheatgerm. Spoon two-thirds of the mixture into the base of the lined cake tin and press flat. Sprinkle the chopped prunes in an even layer over the top then cover with the remaining muesli and syrup mixture.

4 Scatter with the extra dry muesli then bake in a preheated oven, 180°C (350°F, Gas Mark 4), for 25–30 minutes until golden-brown. Leave to cool in the tin.

5 Lift the paper and the muesli mixture out of the tin, cut into 10 bars, then wrap each in kitchen foil or clingfilm. Store in an airtight tin for up to 4 days.

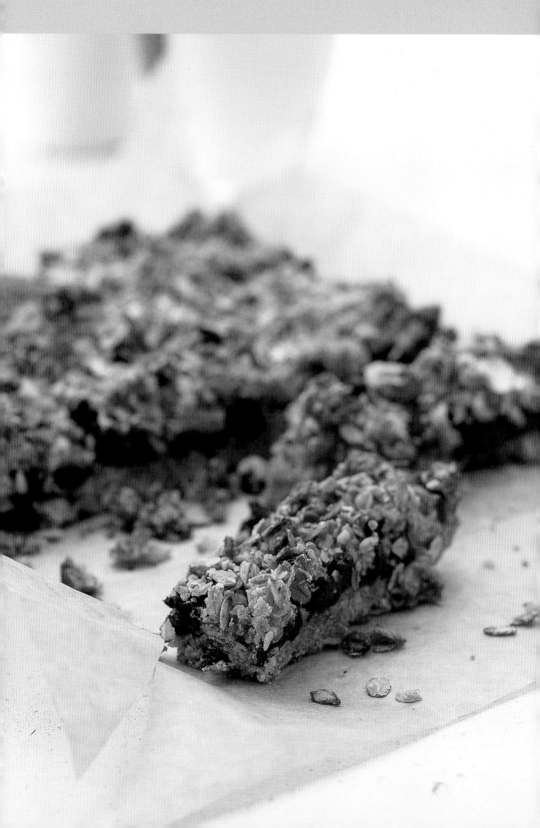

Nutritional values

Kcals 530 (2230 Kj)

fat 15 g

protein 16 g

carbohydrate 88 g

Good source of Vitamin E

Preparation time

25 minutes

Cooking time

25–30 minutes

Serves

6–8

NUTRITIONAL TIP

Dried fruit boosts the iron level of this tasty, high-fibre bread, which is also a moderate source of calcium. Golden linseeds contain lignan, which binds to the body's own oestrogen.

sunflower and fig soda bread

This soda bread is a wonderful treat for a weekend breakfast. Because there is no yeast in the recipe the dough can be mixed and baked immediately without the need for proving, so it's a good standby if you run out of bread.

425 g (14 oz) granary or malthouse flour, plus extra for sprinkling

25 g (1 oz) wheatgerm

50 g (2 oz) sunflower seeds

25 g (1 oz) golden linseeds

1 teaspoon bicarbonate of soda

½ teaspoon salt

125 g (4 oz) light muscovado sugar

200 g (7 oz) ready-to-eat dried figs, roughly chopped

1 teaspoon cream of tartar

200 ml (7 fl oz) semi-skimmed milk

3 tablespoons olive oil

1 egg, beaten

1 Put all the dry ingredients except the cream of tartar in a large bowl then mix in the figs. Stir the cream of tartar into the milk, then add the oil and egg and mix together. Gradually stir this liquid into the dry ingredients to make a soft but not sticky dough.

2 Turn out the dough on to a lightly floured surface and shape it into a circle about 20 cm (8 inches) in diameter.

3 Transfer the round to a lightly greased baking sheet. Cut a large cross in the dough and sprinkle with a little extra flour. Bake in a preheated oven, 200°C (400°F, Gas Mark 6), for 25–30 minutes until well risen and the bread sounds hollow when tapped with your fingertips.

4 Wrap the soda bread in a tea towel to keep it hot and to soften the crust. Cut it into thick slices and serve warm with butter.

Nutritional values

Kcals 195 (815 Kj)

fat 4 g

protein 6 g

carbohydrate 35 g

Excellent source of Vitamin C

Preparation time

20 minutes

Cooking time

Serves

4

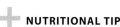 **NUTRITIONAL TIP**

A refreshing start to the day that is packed with Vitamin C and also contains cryptoxanthin, a type of carotenoid. Fromage frais provides calcium.

three-fruit refresher
with banana cream

Make the fruit salad the night before and store it in the refrigerator, then simply mash the banana and mix it into the fromage frais just before serving for a vitality-boosting breakfast.

1 ruby grapefruit

3 oranges

2 kiwifruit, peeled

1 ripe banana

200 g (7 oz) fromage frais

1 tablespoon clear honey

1 Cut the top and bottom off the grapefruit with a serrated knife to reveal the fruit, then cut away the remaining peel and pith. Holding the fruit above a serving bowl, cut between the membranes to release the fruit segments. Repeat the process with the oranges.

2 Cut the kiwifruit in half then into thin wedges. Mix with the citrus fruit. Cover and chill if making in advance.

3 Mash the banana with a fork and stir it into the fromage frais with the honey. Spoon the fruit salad into bowls and serve topped with the banana cream.

Nutritional values

Kcals 240 (1015 Kj)

fat 6 g

protein 12 g

carbohydrate 37 g

Good source of calcium

Preparation time

2 minutes

Cooking time

13–15 minutes

Serves

2–3

NUTRITIONAL TIP

This high-grain porridge provides the ideal balance of starchy foods (two starch portions) to start the day. The dried fruit boosts carotenoids and iron.

mixed grain porridge

This mixed-grain porridge may make true Scots throw up their hands in horror, but it is an easy way to introduce all members of the family to a wider variety of health-promoting grains.

450 ml (¾ pint) semi-skimmed milk

25 g (1 oz) millet grain

25 g (1 oz) barley flakes

25 g (1 oz) oats

TO SERVE
fromage frais

muscovado sugar

ready-to-eat dried fruits, such as apricots and cranberries, chopped

1 Pour the milk into a saucepan, bring to the boil then add the grains.

2 Reduce the heat and simmer for 8–10 minutes, stirring occasionally until thickened and the grains are softened.

3 Spoon into bowls. Top with fromage frais and sprinkle with a little muscovado sugar and chopped ready-to-eat dried fruits.

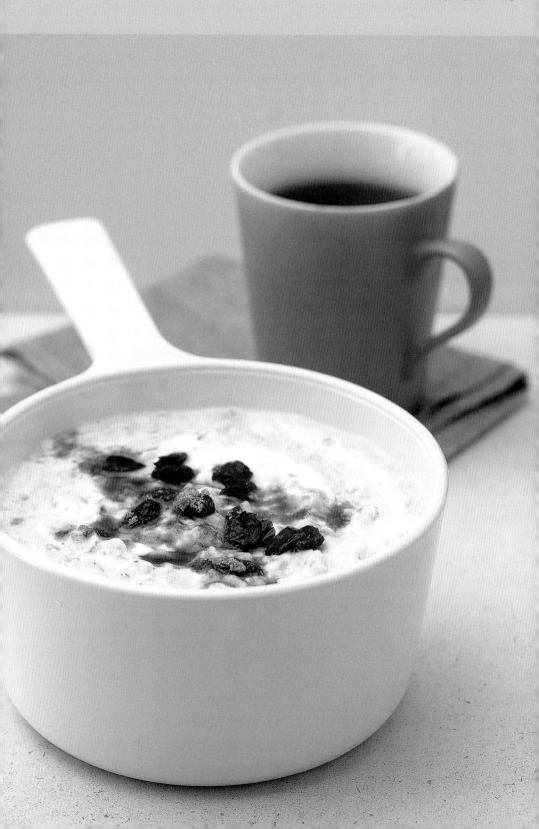

Nutritional values

Kcals 290 (1210 Kj)

fat 14 g

protein 5 g

carbohydrate 38 g

Good source of Vitamin E

Preparation time

3 minutes

Cooking time

10–12 minutes

Serves

6

NUTRITIONAL TIP

The mixed grains, seeds and nuts that form the crunchy topping for the fruit and yogurt give an excellent balance of starchy foods.

honeyed granola

By making your own breakfast cereal you know exactly how much sugar it contains. This crunchy, American-style breakfast topping keeps well in a jar and is delicious sprinkled over sliced fruits and yogurt.

3 tablespoons sunflower oil

3 tablespoons thick honey

2 tablespoons golden linseeds

2 tablespoons sesame seeds

50 g (2 oz) hazelnuts, roughly chopped

50 g (2 oz) barley flakes

50 g (2 oz) rye flakes

50 g (2 oz) millet flakes

1 Warm the oil and honey together in a saucepan then stir in all the remaining ingredients and mix together well.

2 Tip the mixture on to a lightly oiled baking sheet with edges and spread into a thin, even layer. Bake in a preheated oven, 180°C (350°F, Gas Mark 4), for 8–10 minutes until golden-brown, turning and stirring the mixture half way through cooking so that the outer browned edges are moved to the centre and the paler mixture to the outside edges.

3 Leave the toasted mixture to cool then transfer it to a storage jar. Store in a cool place for up to 2 weeks.

Nutritional values

Kcals 185 (780 Kj)

fat 3 g

protein 7 g

carbohydrate 35 g

Good source of carotenoids

Preparation time

20 minutes, plus cooling

Cooking time

5 minutes

Serves

4

NUTRITIONAL TIP

These pretty, layered, fruit-flavoured yogurts are low in fat and a good source of calcium. Adding fresh orange juice, which is rich in vitamin C, helps the absorption of iron from the apricots.

apricot and yogurt layer

Natural fruit sugars sweeten these yogurts to give a healthy mineral-boosting start to the day. The apricot and orange purée will also make a tasty spread for toast or as a cake filling.

150 g (5 oz) ready-to-eat dried apricots, plus extra, cut into strips, to decorate

150 ml (¼ pint) boiling water

juice of 1 orange

250 g (8 oz) natural bio yogurt

2 tablespoons wheatgerm

1 Put the apricots and water in a small saucepan, cover then simmer for 5 minutes until softened. Leave to cool for 15 minutes.

2 Purée the apricots in a liquidizer or food processor with the orange juice until smooth.

3 Mix the yogurt and wheatgerm in a bowl then stir in 2 tablespoons of the apricot purée to sweeten.

4 Divide one-third of the yogurt mixture among 4 x 100 ml (3½ fl oz) glass dishes. Top with half the apricot purée and smooth with a teaspoon to the edges of the dishes.

5 Cover with half the remaining yogurt mixture then the last of the apricot purée. Complete with a final layer of yogurt. Decorate with strips of apricot, if liked. Chill in the refrigerator until required and use within 2 days.

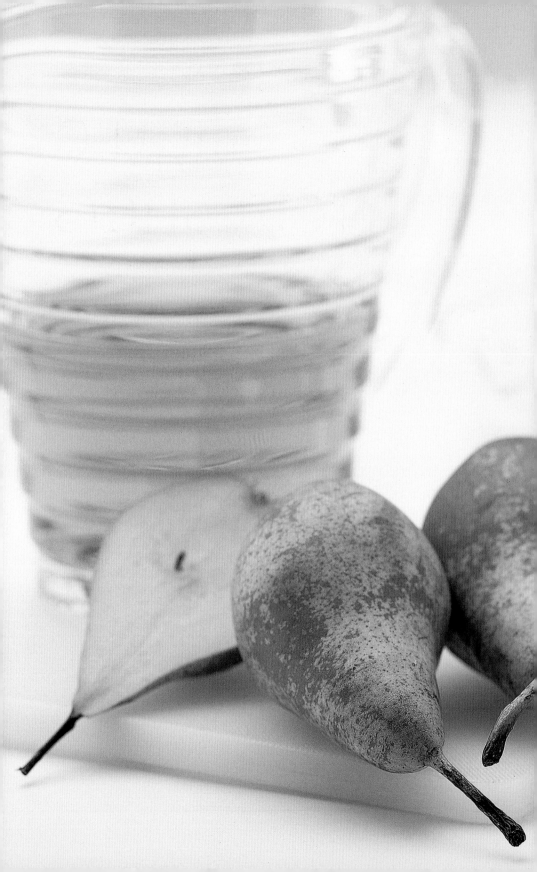

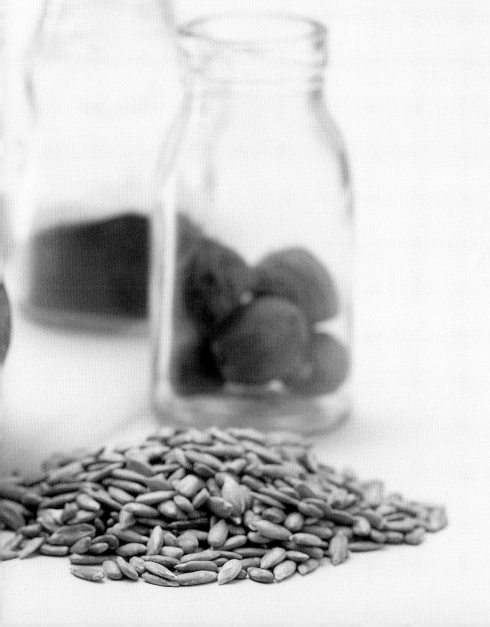

liquid refreshers

Nutritional values

Kcals 180 (780 Kj)

fat 2 g

protein 3 g

carbohydrate 42 g

Good source of carotene

Preparation time

10 minutes

Serves

2

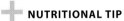 **NUTRITIONAL TIP**

Wonderfully bright and fresh-tasting, this deep pink juice is bursting with Vitamin C and is the perfect start to any day.

watermelon and strawberry blush

Strawberries and limes are both packed with vitamin C, and watermelon contains such a high proportion of water that the finished drink does not need to be diluted. This delicious juice is pure fruit.

1 kg (2 lb) piece of watermelon

200 g (7 oz) strawberries, hulled

juice of 1 lime

1 Use a large spoon to scoop the melon flesh away from the green rind and put it in a liquidizer or food processor goblet. Add the strawberries and blend briefly until it is just mixed.

2 Pour into a sieve set over a large jug then press the pulp through the sieve until only the black seeds remain.

3 Mix the purée with the lime juice then pour into 2 glasses and serve.

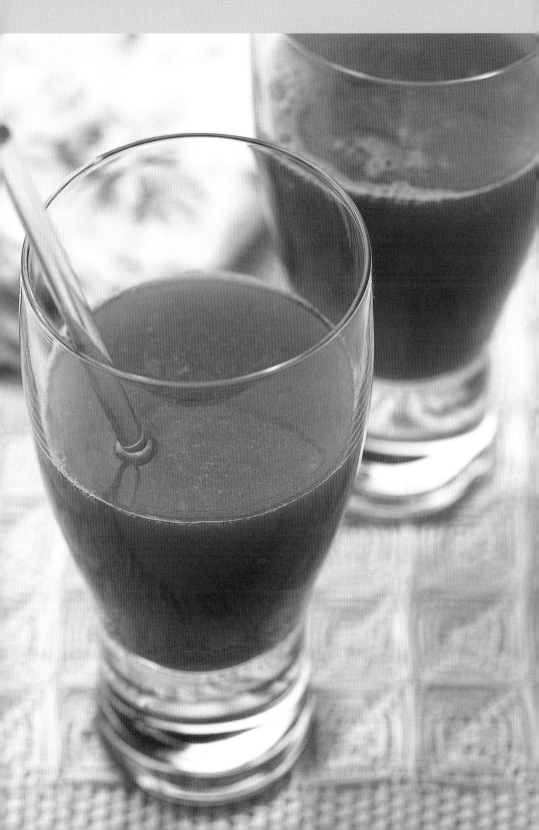

Nutritional values

Kcals 280 (1180 Kj)

fat 15 g

protein 8 g

carbohydrate 30 g

Good source of vitamin E

Preparation time

10 minutes

Serves

2

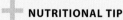 **NUTRITIONAL TIP**

This high-calcium smoothie is also high in fibre. Mild and delicately flavoured, it is a perfect pick-me-up. Hazelnuts contain essential fatty acids and are rich in protein.

spiced pear and hazelnut smoothie

This delicious smoothie is made with the most everyday of ingredients. Rather than toast the hazelnuts every time you make this smoothie, toast a large batch, cool them and store them in a screw-topped jar for up to two weeks.

40 g (1½ oz) hazelnuts

2 ripe pears, peeled, cored and quartered

¼ teaspoon ground cinnamon

150 g (5 oz) natural bio yogurt

150 ml (¼ pint) white grape or apple juice

1 Dry-fry the hazelnuts in a frying pan for 2–3 minutes until lightly browned. Blend them in a liquidizer until finely ground.

2 Add the pears, ground cinnamon and yogurt and blend until smooth. Add the fruit juice and blend briefly until just mixed. Pour into 2 glasses and serve.

Nutritional values

Kcals 310 (1310 Kj)

fat 8 g

protein 7 g

carbohydrate 56 g

Good source of vitamin C

Preparation time

10 minutes

Serves

2

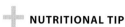 **NUTRITIONAL TIP**

Tofu is an invaluable source of protein for vegetarians and this breakfast smoothie is packed with fibre, vitamin C and vitamin E. Linseeds and tofu contain phytoestrogens.

big breakfast booster

Creamy smooth, this dairy-free drink, packed with natural fruit sugars and protein, makes a satisfying meal in a glass. Linseeds may be a little difficult to find but will be stocked in most health-food shops.

1 tablespoon sunflower seeds

1 tablespoon golden linseeds

1 banana, roughly chopped

4 ready-to-eat dried figs

50 g (2 oz) tofu

450 ml (¾ pint) apple juice

1 Put the seeds in a liquidizer and blend until finely ground.

2 Add the banana, figs, tofu and a little of the fruit juice and blend until smooth.

3 Gradually mix in the remaining fruit juice and blend until frothy. Pour into 2 glasses and serve.

Nutritional values

Kcals 140 (585 Kj)

fat 1 g

protein 2 g

carbohydrate 35 g

Excellent source of carotenoids

Preparation time

10 minutes

Serves

2

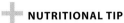 **NUTRITIONAL TIP**

This vibrant juice is packed with carotenoids. These are converted to Vitamin A by the body. They are particularly important for normal tissue growth and as an antioxidant.

gingered apple and carrot juice

An amazingly orange-coloured juice, with just a hint of sweetness, this refreshing drink packs a surprisingly peppery gingered punch. If you are serving this juice to children, reduce the amount of ginger to 1 cm (½ inch).

375 g (12 oz) carrots, scrubbed and cut into chunky pieces

3 apples, cut into chunky pieces

2.5 cm (1 inch) fresh root ginger, peeled

1 Feed the carrot and apple chunks through a juicer with the ginger.

2 Pour the juice into two tumblers and serve.

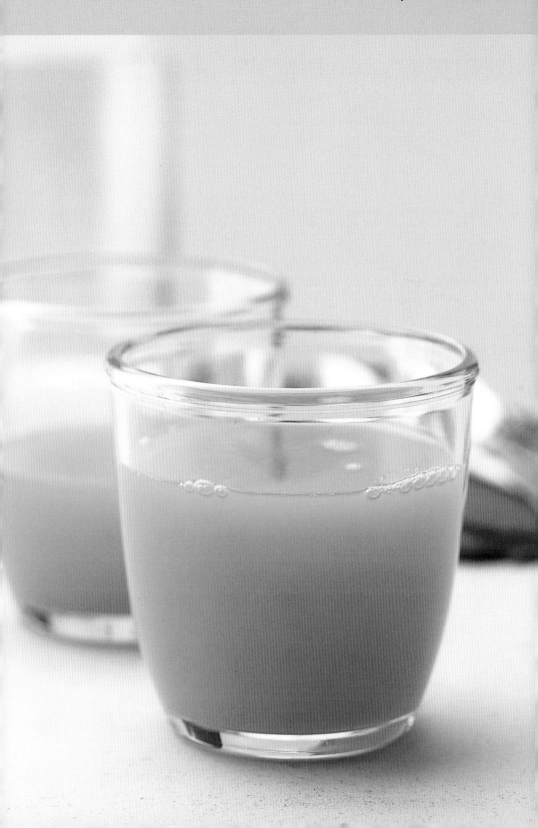

Nutritional values

Kcals 75 (315 Kj)

fat 1 g

protein 2 g

carbohydrate 15 g

Excellent source of vitamin C

Preparation time

15 minutes

Serves

2

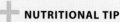 **NUTRITIONAL TIP**

Tomatoes and peppers are good sources of carotenoids and tomatoes are also particularly high in lycopene. This refreshing juice also contains vitamins C and E, both of which are vital antioxidants.

bloody marianna

A 'bloody Mary' without the alcohol, this mixed juice is bursting with vitamins and minerals. This juice will only taste as good as the tomatoes you use, so include those ripened on the vine for extra flavour.

2 celery sticks, plus extra to serve (optional)

¼ cucumber

375 g (12 oz) tomatoes

½ red pepper, cored and deseeded

1 apple

2–3 sprigs of mint

Worcestershire sauce, to taste

Tabasco sauce, to taste

1 Cut all the vegetables and fruit into chunky pieces and then feed them through a juicer with the fresh mint.

2 Stir in the Worcestershire and Tabasco sauces to taste, then pour into 2 glasses half-filled with ice. Serve with celery stick stirrers, if liked.

Nutritional values

Kcals 110 (480 Kj)

fat 1 g

protein 2 g

carbohydrate 26 g

Excellent source of vitamin C

Preparation time

10 minutes

Serves

2

 NUTRITIONAL TIP

A single kiwifruit contains more than the normal daily adult requirement of vitamin C. In addition, it contains potassium, which is needed for the normal function of all the cells in the body.

racing green

This delicious blend of melon, kiwifruit and apple makes a fresh fruity juice. Make sure you buy a green-fleshed melon so that the finished juice is a delicate shade of green.

½ green-fleshed ogen melon

2 kiwifruit, peeled

1 green-skinned dessert apple

1 Cut the fruit into chunky pieces then pass them through a juicer.

2 Half fill two tumblers with ice cubes, pour in the juice and serve.

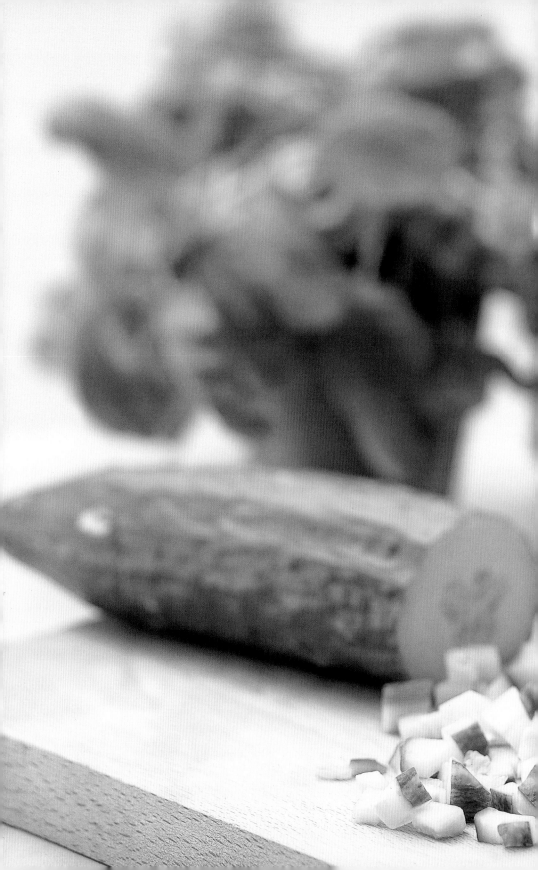

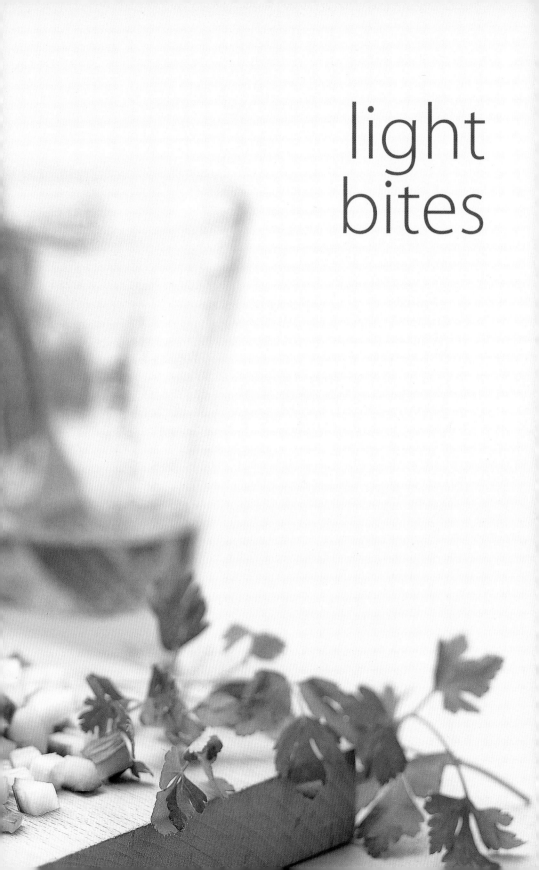

light
bites

Nutritional values

Kcals 240 (1010 Kj)

fat 5 g

protein 40 g

carbohydrate 10 g

Good source of carotenoids

Preparation time

15 minutes

Cooking time

5 minutes

Serves

4

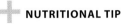 **NUTRITIONAL TIP**

The colourful ingredients in this recipe provide many nutrients, including calcium, magnesium and folate. Mangoes are a particularly good source of the carotenoid cryptoxanthin.

spiced chicken and mango salad

Coronation chicken is a popular dish, but it's made with a mayonnaise dressing that's packed with calories and fat. This healthier version keeps the fat content low by using a natural yogurt dressing and steaming the chicken.

4 boneless, skinless chicken breasts, about 150 g (5 oz) each

6 teaspoons mild curry paste

juice of 1 lemon

150 g (5 oz) natural bio yogurt

1 mango

50 g (2 oz) watercress

½ cucumber, diced

½ red onion, chopped

½ iceberg lettuce

1 Rinse the chicken breasts with cold water, drain well and cut into long, thin slices. Put 4 teaspoons of the curry paste in a plastic bag with the lemon juice and mix together by squeezing the bag. Add the chicken and toss together.

2 Half-fill the base of a steamer with water and bring to the boil. Place the chicken in the top of the steamer in a single layer, cover and steam for 5 minutes until thoroughly cooked. Test with a knife – the juices will run clear when done.

3 Meanwhile, mix the remaining curry paste in a bowl with the yogurt.

4 Cut a thick slice off either side of the mango to reveal the large, flat stone. Trim the flesh away from the stone, then remove the peel and cut the flesh into bite-sized chunks.

5 Rinse the watercress with cold water and tear it into bite-sized pieces. Add to the yogurt dressing with the cucumber, red onion and mango and toss together gently.

6 Tear the lettuce into pieces, divide it among 4 plates, spoon the mango mixture on top and complete with the warm chicken strips.

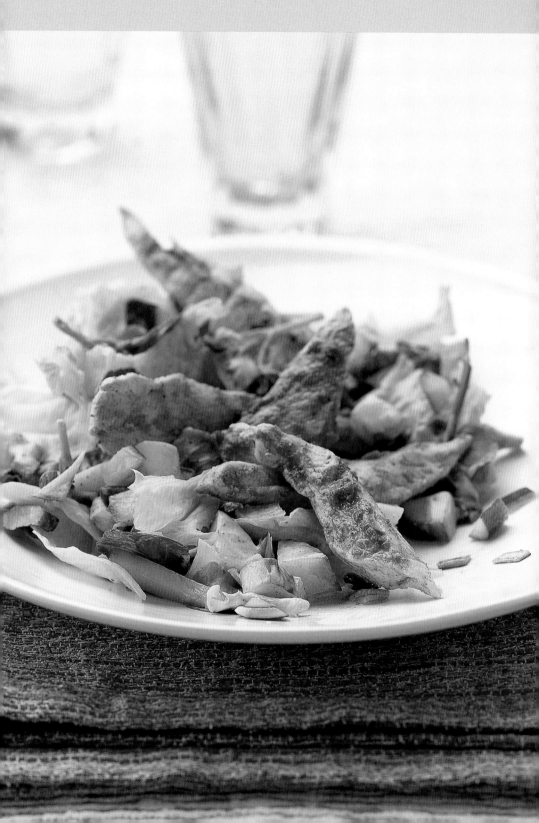

Nutritional values

Kcals 170 (710 Kj)

fat 11 g

protein 11 g

carbohydrate 8 g

Good source of fibre

Preparation time

15 minutes

Cooking time

2–3 minutes

Serves

4

NUTRITIONAL TIP

Soya beans are rich in phytoestrogens as well as all the essential amino acids. This high-protein, high-fibre snack also contains folate.

hummus

Low in fat and packed with protein, this Greek-style spread makes both a great dip for vegetable crudités and a sandwich filler with salad. It will keep well in the refrigerator for 2–3 days.

3 tablespoons sesame seeds

250 g (8 oz) cooked soya beans

2 garlic cloves, crushed

¼ onion (optional)

juice of 1 lemon

5 tablespoons semi-skimmed milk

1 tablespoon olive oil (optional)

1 teaspoon clear honey

salt and pepper

TO GARNISH
paprika, for sprinkling

black olives

TO SERVE
carrot, celery and cucumber sticks

warm wholemeal pitta bread, cut into strips

1 Dry-fry the sesame seeds over a gentle heat until lightly toasted then grind in a liquidizer or food processor.

2 Add the remaining ingredients and blend the mixture to a smooth paste. Spoon into a serving bowl, sprinkle with a little paprika and top with a few black olives.

3 Place the bowl on a large plate and surround it with vegetable sticks and strips of pitta bread.

Nutritional values

Kcals 300 (1250 Kj)

fat 8 g

protein 25 g

carbohydrate 32 g

Excellent source of fibre

Preparation time

10 minutes

Cooking time

4 minutes

Serves

4

 NUTRITIONAL TIP

The colourful combination of vegetables and beans here provides phytoestrogens. Frozen and canned pulses are just as good nutritionally as fresh, but choose ones canned without salt and sugar if possible.

tuna and mixed bean salad

Quick and easy to put together, a mixed bean salad makes an ideal lunch served with French wholegrain bread. This colourful version is made with a combination of fresh, canned and frozen beans.

75 g (3 oz) French beans

200 g (7 oz) frozen broad beans

125 g (4 oz) frozen sweetcorn

2 tablespoons olive oil

2 tablespoons red wine vinegar

1 teaspoon wholegrain mustard

410 g (13¼ oz) can red kidney beans, drained and rinsed

185 g (6¼ oz) can tuna in springwater, drained and flaked

½ red onion, thinly sliced

salt and pepper

1 Bring a saucepan of water to the boil, add the French beans and cook for 2 minutes. Add the frozen broad beans and sweetcorn and cook for 2 more minutes. Tip into a colander, drain well, rinse with cold water and drain again.

2 Mix the oil, vinegar, mustard and salt and pepper together in a bowl.

3 Stir in the kidney beans. Add the flaked tuna and the red onion and toss together lightly.

Nutritional values

Kcals 205 (845 Kj)

fat 13 g

protein 12 g

carbohydrate 10 mg

Excellent source of vitamin C

Preparation time

10 minutes

Cooking time

8 minutes

Serves

4

NUTRITIONAL TIP

Preserve the vitamin C content of vegetables by lightly steaming or stir-frying them. As well as providing vitamin C, broccoli is a good source of the bioactive compound isothiocyanate.

Italian broccoli and egg salad

The addition of a tangy lemon and caper dressing subtly flavoured with delicate fresh tarragon really transforms plain steamed broccoli and leeks into a light gourmet meal.

4 eggs

300 g (10 oz) broccoli

2 small leeks (about 300 g/ 10 oz), trimmed, slit and well rinsed

juice of 1 lemon

2 tablespoons olive oil

2 teaspoons clear honey

1 tablespoon capers, well drained

2 tablespoons chopped fresh tarragon

salt and pepper

sprigs of tarragon, to garnish (optional)

wholemeal bread, to serve

1 Half-fill the base of a steamer with water, add the eggs and bring to the boil. Cover with the steamer top and simmer for 8 minutes until hard-boiled.

2 Meanwhile, cut the broccoli into florets and thickly slice the broccoli stems and the leeks. Add the broccoli to the top of the steamer, cook for 3 minutes, add the leeks and cook for another 2 minutes.

3 Mix the remaining ingredients together in a salad bowl to make the dressing.

4 Crack the hard-boiled eggs, cool them quickly under running water, then remove the shells and roughly chop the eggs.

5 Add the broccoli and leeks to the dressing, toss together and sprinkle with the chopped eggs. Garnish with sprigs of extra tarragon if liked and serve warm with thickly sliced wholemeal bread.

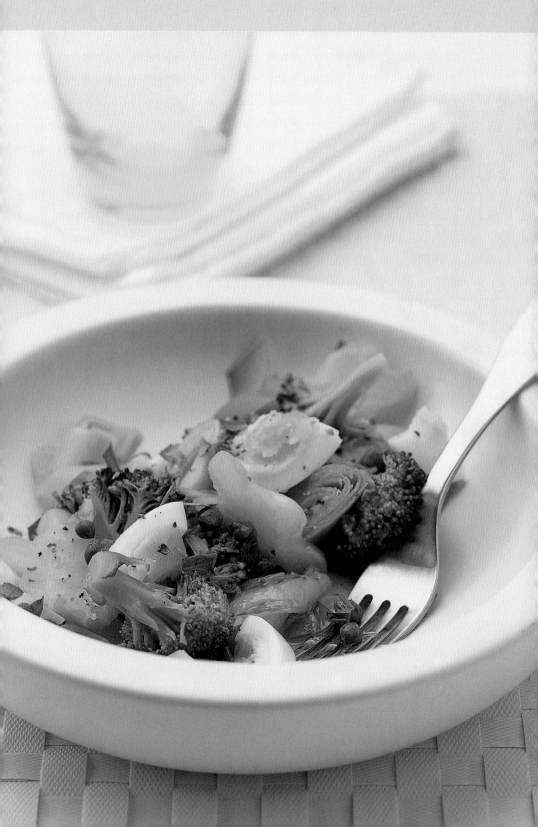

Nutritional values

Kcals 100 (415 Kj)

fat 2 g

protein 6 g

carbohydrate 17 g

Good source of carotene

Preparation time

10 minutes

Cooking time

Serves

4

＋ NUTRITIONAL TIP

A colourful salad that is a good source of vitamin C with a virtually fat-free dressing. It provides the daily requirement for beta-carotene in one serving.

carrot and sprouting bean salad

Made in minutes, this salad can be served as a sandwich filling spooned into wholemeal rolls with sliced chicken or with cheese, tomatoes and cucumber or one of a selection of different salads for dinner.

juice of 1 orange

2 teaspoons wholegrain mustard

1 teaspoon clear honey

300 g (10 oz) carrots, coarsely grated

250 g (8 oz) mixed sprouting seeds, rinsed and well drained

salt and pepper

1 Put the orange juice, mustard, honey and salt and pepper in a salad bowl and fork together.

2 Stir the grated carrots into the dressing with the sprouting seeds.

Nutritional values

Kcals 185 (775 Kj)

fat 6 g

protein 6 g

carbohydrate 29 g

Excellent source of carotene

Preparation time

25 minutes

Cooking time

37 minutes

Serves

6

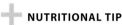 **NUTRITIONAL TIP**

Perfect for a winter lunch, this warming soup is packed with a variety of nutrients including carotenoids, magnesium and calcium. If using a stock cube, make sure you choose one that it is low in salt.

carrot and pepperpot soup

This is an amazingly vibrantly coloured, velvety soup with a delicate flavour. It is ideal for storing in the freezer in handy individual servings, ready to microwave. Serve on its own with warmed bread or topped with low-fat croûtons.

1 tablespoon olive oil

1 onion, chopped

500 g (1 lb) carrots, diced

1 red pepper, cored, deseeded and diced

1.2 litres (2 pints) vegetable stock

PESTO CROÛTONS
6 slices of wholemeal French stick

3 teaspoons pesto

freshly grated Parmesan cheese (optional)

1 Heat the oil in a saucepan, add the onion and cook gently for 5 minutes until softened.

2 Add the carrots and red pepper and cook for 2 minutes. Pour in the stock, bring to the boil, then cover and simmer for 30 minutes until the vegetables are tender.

3 Purée the vegetables and stock in batches in a liquidizer or food processor. Pour back into the saucepan and reheat.

4 Meanwhile, lightly toast the bread on both sides then spread with the pesto. Ladle the soup into bowls, float the croûtons on top and sprinkle with Parmesan, if using.

Nutritional values

Kcals 72 (300 Kj)

fat 5 g

protein 6 g

carbohydrate 2 g

Good source of iron

Preparation time

15 minutes

Cooking time

20 minutes

Serves

12

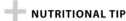 **NUTRITIONAL TIP**

Tasty and very moreish, these snacks are packed with nutrients, including iron, beta-carotene and calcium. Balance the meal with wholemeal pitta bread and a fresh green salad.

broccoli and spinach eggah

Popular in the Middle East, eggah, which is baked and served as a mezze dish, is rather like a quiche without the pastry. Rather than making one large dish, these tiny eggahs have been baked in the individual sections of a deep muffin tin.

125 g (4 oz) broccoli

100 g (3½ oz) young spinach leaves

6 eggs

300 ml (½ pint) semi-skimmed milk

2 tablespoons grated Parmesan cheese

large pinch of ground nutmeg

salt and pepper

warm wholemeal pitta bread, to serve

1 Cut the broccoli into small florets and thickly slice the stems. Put in a steamer set over boiling water. Cover and cook for 3 minutes. Add the spinach and cook for 1 minute more or until just wilted.

2 Beat the eggs, milk, Parmesan, nutmeg and a little salt and pepper together in a jug. Divide the broccoli and spinach among the sections of a lightly oiled deep 12-hole muffin tin, then cover with the egg mixture.

3 Bake in a preheated oven, 190°C (375°F, Gas Mark 5), for about 15 minutes until lightly browned, well risen and the egg mixture has set. Leave in the tin for 1–2 minutes, then loosen the edges with a knife and turn out. Serve 2–3 per person with warmed wholemeal pitta bread.

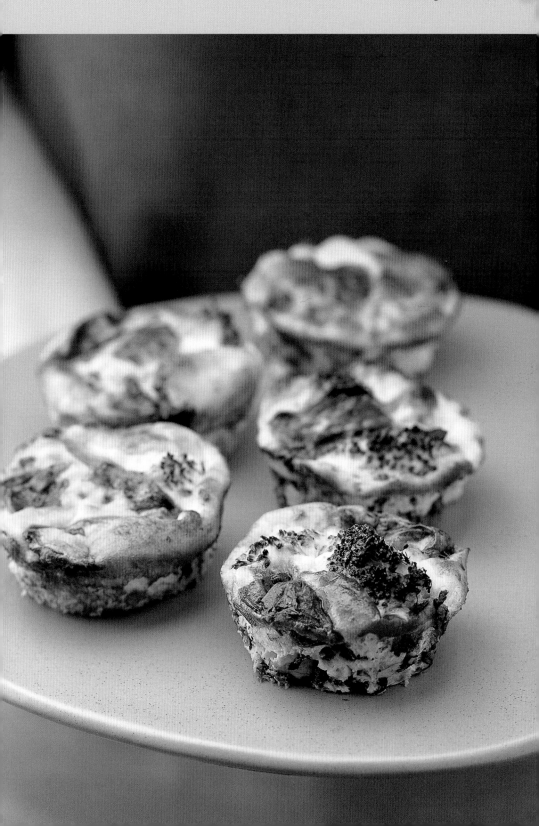

Nutritional values

Kcals 210 (890 Kj)

fat 4 g

protein 20 g

carbohydrate 26 g

Preparation time

15 minutes

Cooking time

7 minutes

Serves

4

NUTRITIONAL TIP

An excellent balance is provided by this light soup, which is low in fat and high in carbohydrate. Fish sauce and soy sauce are both high in salt, but as long as they are used in small amounts they can be included in the diet.

Thai prawn broth

This refreshing clear broth is speckled with shiitake mushrooms, red pepper, pak choi and prawns and flavoured with kaffir lime and coriander leaves. If serving to vegetarians, leave out the prawns and fish sauce.

1.2 litres (2 pints) vegetable stock

2 teaspoons Thai red curry paste

4 dried kaffir lime leaves, torn into pieces

4 teaspoons fish sauce

2 spring onions, sliced

150 g (5 oz) shiitake mushrooms, sliced

125 g (4 oz) soba (Japanese noodles)

½ red pepper, cored, deseeded and diced

125 g (4 oz) pak choi, thinly sliced

250 g (8 oz) frozen prawns, defrosted and rinsed

small bunch of coriander leaves, torn into pieces

1 Pour the stock into a saucepan, add the curry paste, lime leaves, fish sauce, onions and mushrooms. Bring to the boil and simmer for 5 minutes.

2 Bring a separate pan of water to the boil, add the noodles and cook for 3 minutes.

3 Add the remaining ingredients to the soup and cook for 2 minutes until piping hot.

4 Drain the noodles, rinse with fresh hot water and spoon into the base of 4 bowls. Ladle the hot prawn broth over the top and serve immediately.

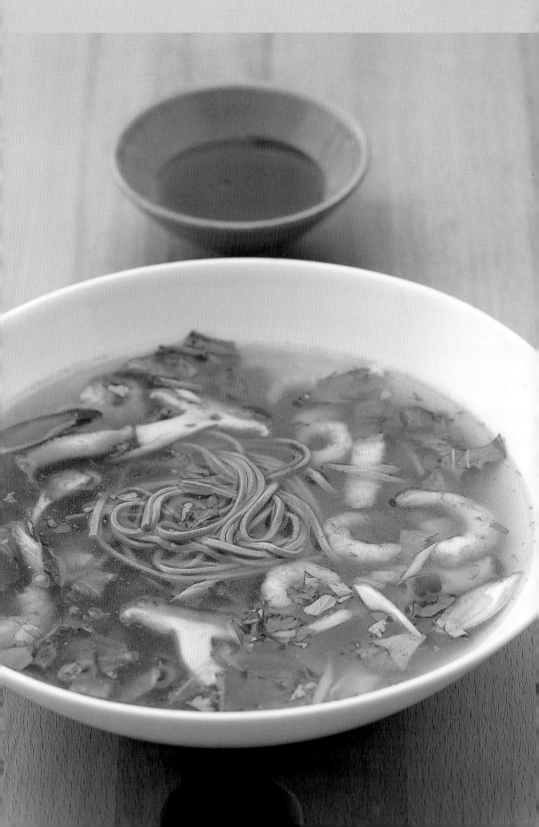

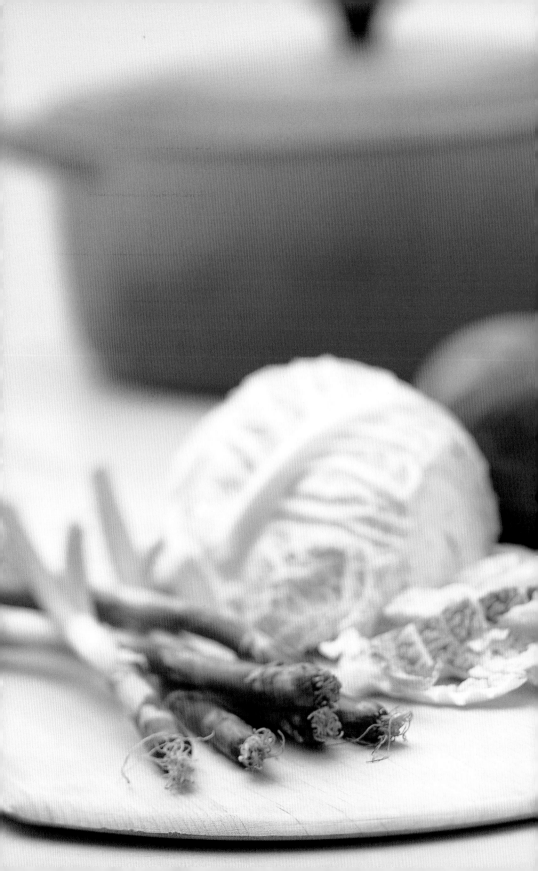

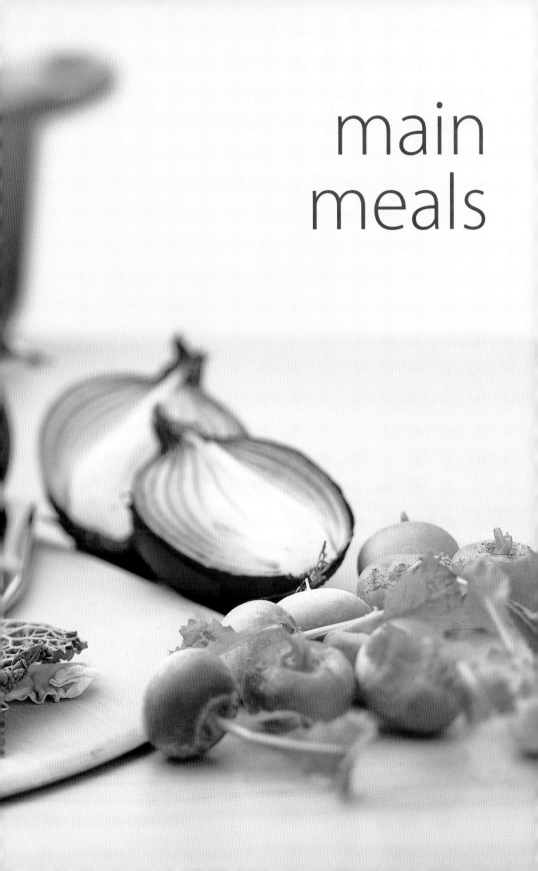

main
meals

Nutritional values
Kcals 750 (3130 Kj)
fat 41 g
protein 52 g
carbohydrate 46 g
Good source of folate

Preparation time
30 minutes
Cooking time
1 hour 20 minutes
Serves
4–5

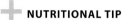 **NUTRITIONAL TIP**
A high-fibre dish that is packed with iron and beta-carotene. Boost vitamin C levels by stirring the juice of an orange into the strained gravy just before serving.

roast chicken
with mixed spiced roots

A roast dinner is popular with all ages but can be laden with fat. Cut down on the oil by tossing the vegetables in a plastic bag of oil. If you carve the chicken thinly there will be enough left for a sandwich or salad for lunch the next day.

1.5 kg (3 lb) oven-ready chicken

2 teaspoons coriander seeds

1 teaspoon fennel seeds

1 teaspoon cumin seeds

2 tablespoons olive oil

½ teaspoon turmeric

½ teaspoon paprika

2 parsnips

2 large carrots

2 sweet potatoes

1 large onion

8 garlic cloves, unpeeled

2 tablespoons plain flour

600 ml (1 pint) chicken stock

coriander leaves, to garnish

1 Remove any giblets and rinse the chicken inside and out with cold water. Drain and place it in a large roasting tin.

2 Crush the seeds and put them in a large plastic bag with the oil and ground spice. Shake until well mixed. Spoon a little of the mixture over the chicken breast, then cover with foil.

3 Roast the chicken in a preheated oven, 190°C (375°F, Gas Mark 5), for 1 hour and 20 minutes.

4 Cut the vegetables into large chunks, add to the bag of spiced oil and toss. Add to the roasting tin after 20 minutes of cooking the chicken, tucking some garlic cloves between the chicken legs and adding the rest to the vegetables. Cook for 1 hour until golden, turning the vegetables after 30 minutes and removing the foil from the chicken at this point.

5 Transfer the chicken and vegetables from the roasting tin to a large serving plate and keep warm. Garnish with coriander. Drain the fat from the meat juices and stir in the flour. To make the gravy, put the roasting tin on the hob and cook for 1 minute, stirring. Gradually stir in the stock and bring to the boil. Strain into a jug and serve immediately.

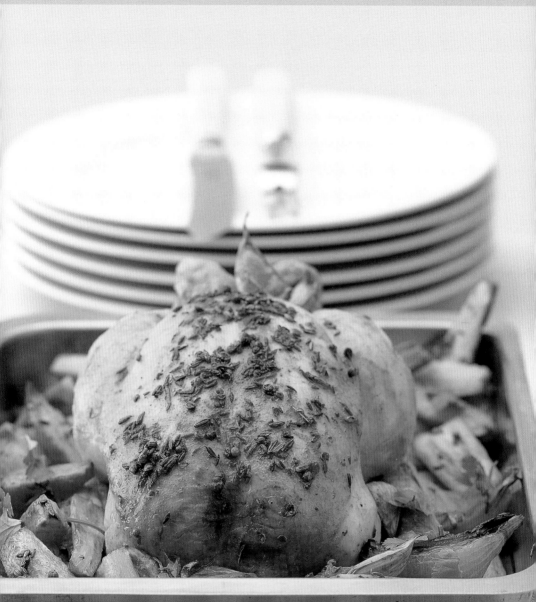

Nutritional values

Kcals 640 (2280 Kj)

fat 3 g

protein 45 g

carbohydrate 86 g

Good source of iron

Preparation time

25 minutes

Cooking time

12–17 minutes

Serves

4

+ NUTRITIONAL TIP

Exceptionally low in fat, this dish provides over half of its energy from carbohydrate – just the right balance. Bulgar wheat is unsuitable for people on a gluten-free diet.

citrus chicken with fruited bulgar

Bulgar wheat takes half the time of brown rice to cook and makes a nutty base for this Moroccan-style spiced pilaf studded with chopped apricots, dates and sultanas, and topped with citrus-steamed chicken breasts.

900 ml (1¹⁄₂ pints) chicken stock

¹⁄₄ teaspoon ground cinnamon

¹⁄₄ teaspoon ground nutmeg or allspice

250 g (8 oz) bulgar wheat

4 boneless, skinless chicken breasts, about 150 g (5 oz) each

grated rind of ¹⁄₂ lemon

grated rind of ¹⁄₂ orange

125 g (4 oz) ready-to-eat dried apricots

75 g (3 oz) stoned dates, chopped

75 g (3 oz) sultanas

juice of 1 orange

salt and pepper

small bunch of fresh coriander or basil, torn, to garnish

1 Pour the stock into the base of a steamer and add the ground spices and bulgar wheat.

2 Rinse the chicken breasts with cold water, drain them, then place in the steamer top and sprinkle with the lemon and orange rind and a little salt and pepper.

3 Bring the stock to the boil, put the steamer top in place, cover with a lid and cook for 10 minutes until the chicken is thoroughly cooked and the bulgar is tender. Remove the steamer top and cook the bulgar for a few extra minutes if needed.

4 Stir the dried fruits and orange juice into the bulgar then spoon the bulgar and any stock on to 4 plates. Slice the chicken pieces, arrange over the bulgar and sprinkle with torn herb leaves to garnish. Serve with a watercress and rocket salad.

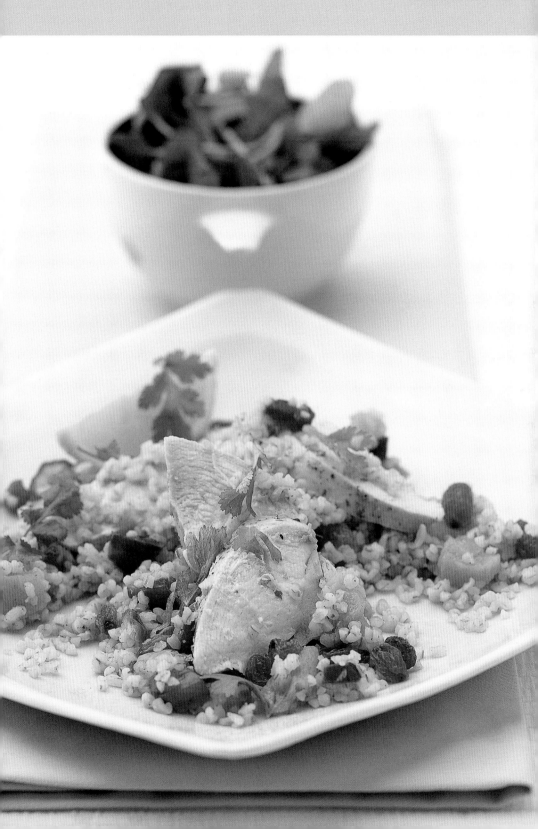

Nutritional values

Kcals 230 (980 Kj)

fat 7 g

protein 37 g

carbohydrate 5 g

Good source of selenium

Preparation time

10 minutes

Cooking time

4–5 minutes

Serves

4

NUTRITIONAL TIP

Tuna is a meaty fish, ideal for winning round those who usually dislike fish. It contains selenium, omega-3 fatty acids, vitamins A, B12 and B3, folate and iron. Fennel is rich in phytoestrogens.

quick tuna and fennel stew

Low in calories and high in protein and minerals, this supper dish is simplicity itself – a perfect recipe to make after a hectic day at work. Serve with a rocket salad and new potatoes.

4 tuna steaks, about 150 g (5 oz) each

4 baby fennel or 1 large bulb, about 175 g (6 oz) total weight, sliced

425 g (14 oz) tomatoes, skinned and diced

2 teaspoons tomato purée

grated rind of 1 lemon

3 tablespoons chopped fresh parsley or basil

salt and pepper

lemon wedges, to garnish

1 Cut the tuna into chunks about 5 cm (2 inches) square and put them in a frying pan. Top with the fennel and tomatoes and sprinkle with a little salt and pepper.

2 Cover and cook over a medium heat for 2 minutes. Lift the lid, turn the pieces of tuna over and stir the tomato purée into the juices. Cover and cook for 2–3 minutes until the tuna is cooked through.

3 Spoon on to 4 plates, sprinkle with the lemon rind and herbs, add the lemon wedges and serve.

Nutritional values

Kcals 450 (1875 Kj)

fat 34 g

protein 35 g

carbohydrate 3 g

Good source of vitamin E

Preparation time

20 minutes, plus

marinating

Cooking time

13–14 minutes

Serves 4

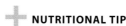 **NUTRITIONAL TIP**

Avocados are a rich source of vitamin E and also contain vitamin C (both are good antioxidants), vitamin B6 and potassium. Avocados are high in fat, however, so eat in moderation.

warm salmon and sesame salad

Crisp crunchy salad leaves mixed with lime, avocado and toasted sesame seeds makes an orientally inspired salad that complements baked salmon perfectly. You could add bean sprouts in place of the watercress, rocket and spinach salad.

4 salmon steaks, about 150 g (5 oz) each

2 tablespoons light soy sauce

4 tablespoons sesame seeds

2 small avocados

juice of 2 limes

½ iceberg lettuce, shredded into bite-sized pieces

125 g (4 oz) bag mixed watercress, spinach and rocket salad

½ cucumber, diced

freshly ground black pepper

1 Rinse the salmon steaks with cold water, drain and put them on a plate. Spoon over half the soy sauce and leave to stand for 15 minutes.

2 Dry-fry the sesame seeds for 3–4 minutes until lightly toasted, remove from the heat, add the remaining soy sauce and quickly cover with a lid. Leave to cool.

3 Place the salmon pieces on a large piece of foil and pour any soy sauce remaining on the plate over the fish. Wrap the salmon loosely in the foil and seal the edges together well. Place on a baking sheet and cook in a preheated oven, 180°C (350°F, Gas Mark 4), for 10 minutes, until the fish flakes when pressed with a knife and the flakes are the same colour throughout.

4 Meanwhile, halve, stone and peel the avocados. Slice and toss them in the lime juice.

5 Place all the salad leaves and cucumber in a large bowl, add the avocado, toasted sesame seeds and a little pepper and toss together. Spoon on to plates and top with the cooked salmon. Serve immediately.

Nutritional values

Kcals 370 (1560 Kj)

fat 7 g

protein 48 g

carbohydrate 30 g

Good source of iron

Preparation time

25 minutes

Cooking time

1 hour 25–28 minutes

Serves

4–5

＋ NUTRITIONAL TIP

Beef is rich in protein, iron and vitamin B12, but aim to keep portion sizes to 80 g (3¼oz), about 2 thin slices (or balance with a meat-free day). The meat is cooked slowly here to avoid the formation of heterocyclic aromatic amines.

one-pot beef

Keep both your fat intake and the washing-up to a minimum by braising a joint of topside together with the accompanying vegetables in one casserole in a well-flavoured gravy.

1 onion, sliced

750 g (1½ lb) topside of beef, trimmed of fat

4 small baking potatoes, peeled and quartered

250 g (8 oz) baby carrots

250 g (8 oz) parsnips, cut into chunks

50 g (2 oz) pearl barley

2 bay leaves

900 ml (1½ pints) beef or chicken stock

1 tablespoon tomato purée

1 teaspoon wholegrain mustard

50 g (5 oz) baby turnips, scrubbed

100 g (3½ oz) green beans

2 baby cabbages, quartered

salt and pepper

1 tablespoon cornflour mixed with a little water

1 Put the onion in the centre of a flameproof casserole dish and stand the beef joint on top. Add the potatoes, carrots and parsnips to the casserole with the pearl barley and bay leaves.

2 Pour the stock into the casserole and add the tomato purée, mustard and salt and pepper. Bring to the boil on the hob then cover and transfer to a preheated oven, 160°C (325°F, Gas Mark 3), and cook for 1¼ hours.

3 Lift the beef out of the casserole, put it on a plate and wrap it in foil to keep warm. Add the turnips to the casserole, cover and simmer on the hob for 5 minutes. Add the green vegetables and cook for a further 5–8 minutes until just tender and still bright green. Stir in the cornflour mix and cook for 1 minute.

4 Thinly slice the beef and arrange on plates. Lift the vegetables out of the pan with a slotted spoon and arrange them around the beef. Spoon the gravy, onions and pearl barley over the meat.

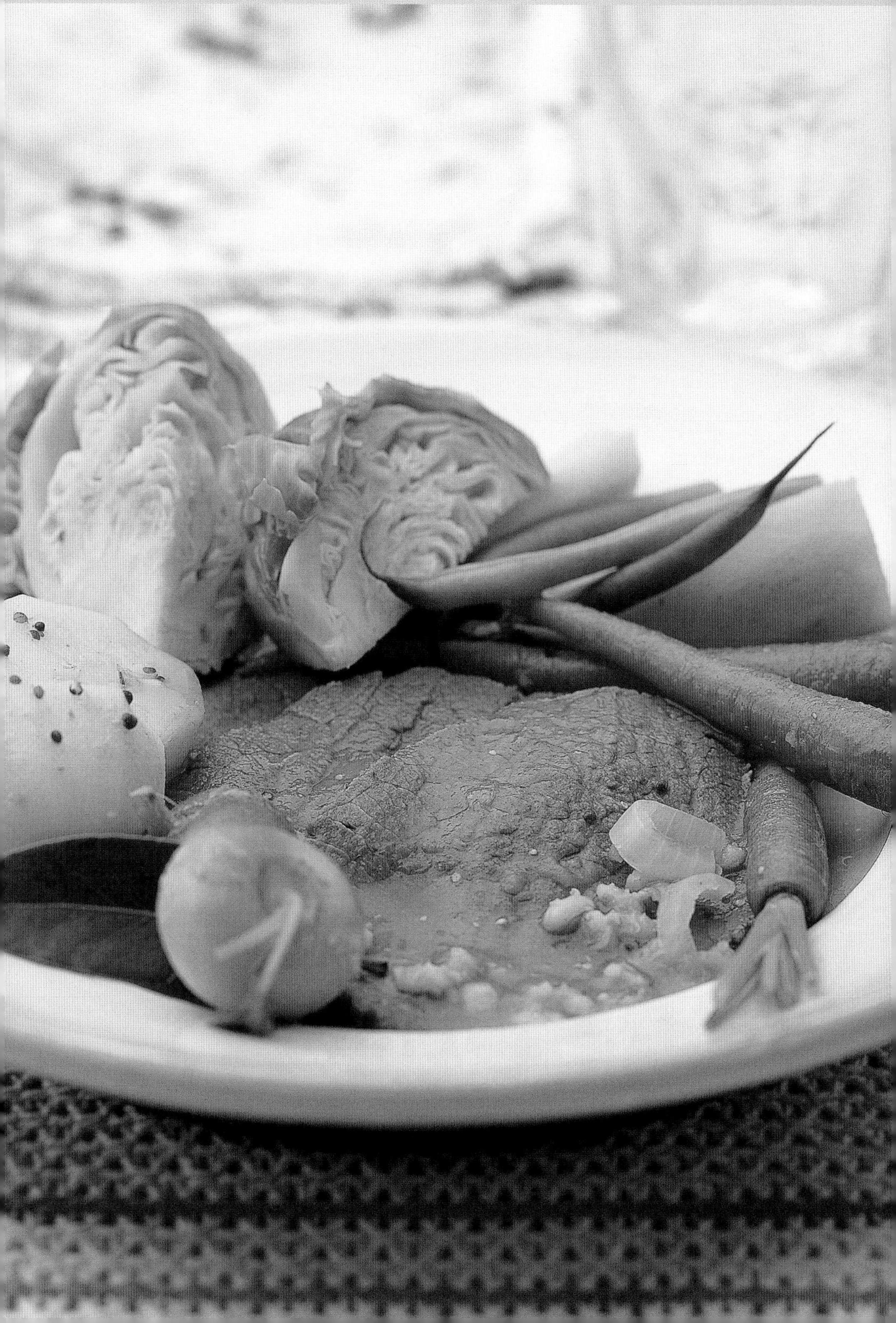

Nutritional values

Kcals 275 (1150 Kj)

fat 12 g

protein 22 g

carbohydrate 21 g

Good source of iron

Preparation time

22 minutes

Cooking time

23 minutes

Serves

4

NUTRITIONAL TIP

This meat dish remains within the recommended portion size and provides fibre, iron and zinc. Using millet instead of breadcrumbs makes the sausages suitable even for those on a gluten-free diet.

pork, prune and leek sausages

Rather than banish sausages from a healthy-eating programme, reduce the amounts of fat by making your own with lean minced pork (or chicken or turkey), steamed leeks and diced prunes, and oven-baking rather than frying them.

150 g (5 oz) leeks, rinsed and diced

375 g (12 oz) lean minced pork

50 g (2 oz) millet flakes

100 g (3½ oz) ready-to-eat pitted prunes, chopped

1 egg yolk

large pinch of ground nutmeg

4 tomatoes, halved

salt and pepper

1 Cook the leeks in the top of a steamer for 3 minutes until just tender.

2 Mix the minced pork in a bowl with the millet flakes, prunes, egg yolk, nutmeg and a little salt and pepper, then stir in the leeks.

3 Spoon the mixture into 8 mounds on a chopping board and shape each into a 10 cm (4 inch) long sausage with wetted hands.

4 Put the sausages in a roasting tin in a preheated oven, 190°C (375°F, Gas Mark 5), and cook for 10 minutes. Add the tomatoes and cook for 10 more minutes until the sausages are golden and the tomatoes are hot. Spoon on to plates and serve immediately, with a green salad if liked.

Nutritional values

Kcals 615 (2570 Kj)

fat 32 g

protein 40 g

carbohydrate 43 g

Good source of selenium

Preparation time

15 minutes

Cooking time

27–30 minutes

Serves

4

✛ NUTRITIONAL NOTES

Everyone loves mashed potato, but sweet potato contains beta-carotene, calcium, magnesium and potassium, plus folic acid and vitamins C and E and so is nutritionally better than ordinary potato.

soused mackerel
with parsnip and chilli mash

Sousing is a traditional method of cooking with vinegar that is rather forgotten about in modern times. Originally cooked in a saucepan, this version is baked in a foil packet so that there is minimal washing up.

500 g (1 lb) sweet potatoes, cut into large dice

425 g (14 oz) parsnips, cut into large dice

4 mackerel fillets cut from 2 large mackerel, about 750 g (1½ lb) total weight

50 g (2 oz) leek, rinsed and thinly sliced

1 carrot, thinly sliced

1 celery stick, sliced

1 tablespoon white wine vinegar

150 ml (¼ pint) hot fish stock

4–5 tablespoons semi-skimmed milk

1 teaspoon chopped red chilli

salt and pepper

steamed green vegetables, to serve

1 Put the sweet potatoes and parsnips into the top of a steamer, add water to the base and bring to the boil. Cover and simmer for 12–15 minutes until tender.

2 Meanwhile, rinse the mackerel fillets with cold water, drain and put on a large sheet of foil set on a shallow baking tray. Cover with the vegetables. Mix the vinegar with the stock and salt and pepper and pour over the fish.

3 Cover with a second piece of foil, twist the edges to seal then cook in a preheated oven, 160°C (325°F, Gas Mark 3), for 15 minutes until the fish flakes easily when pressed with a knife.

4 Drain and mash the sweet potato and parsnip with the milk and chilli. Spoon on to 4 plates and arrange the mackerel by the side. Serve with steamed green vegetables.

Nutritional values

Kcals 315 (1325 Kj)

fat 11 g

protein 41 g

carbohydrate 13 g

Good source of vitamin E

Preparation time

25 minutes

Cooking time

13–16 minutes

Serves

4

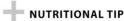 **NUTRITIONAL TIP**

The low fat halibut provides an ideal base for this tasty crust. The topping contains protective compounds such as lycopene from the tomatoes and terpenoid from the lemon rind.

baked halibut with an olive crust

This dish can be prepared in advance, then baked when required for effortless entertaining or a smart family supper. Don't be tempted to use sun-dried tomatoes packed 'dry' in case they burn during cooking.

40 g (1½ oz) pitted black olives, chopped

50 g (2 oz) sun-dried tomatoes in oil, well drained and chopped

grated rind and juice of 1 lemon

4 tablespoons fresh wholemeal breadcrumbs

4 halibut steaks, about 175 g (6 oz) each and 2 cm (¾ inch) thick

salt and pepper

rocket, olive and lemon salad, to serve

1 Put the chopped olives and sun-dried tomatoes in a bowl with the lemon rind, half the juice, the breadcrumbs and a little salt and pepper and mix together.

2 Rinse the fish steaks with cold water, drain and place in a shallow ovenproof dish. Drizzle with the remaining lemon juice then spoon the olive mixture on top.

3 Bake, uncovered, in a preheated oven, 180°C (350°F, Gas Mark 4), for 13–16 minutes until the topping is crisp and the fish is cooked through. Serve with a rocket, olive and lemon salad.

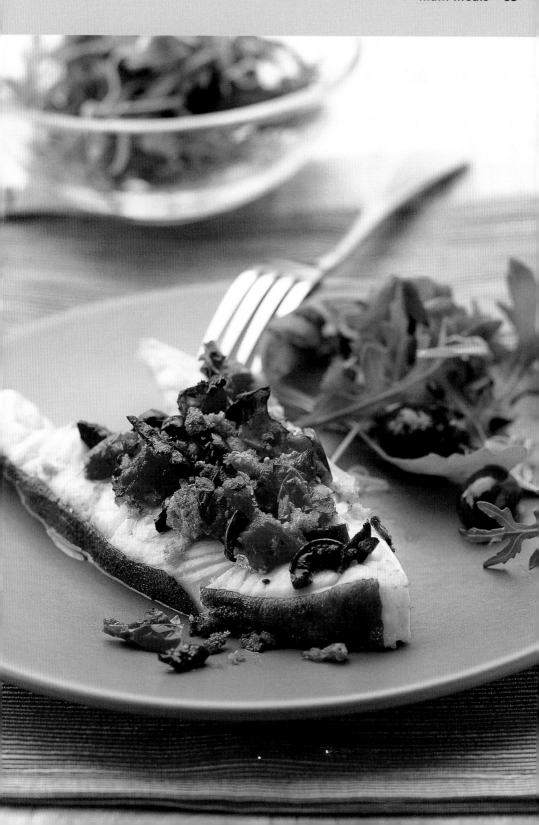

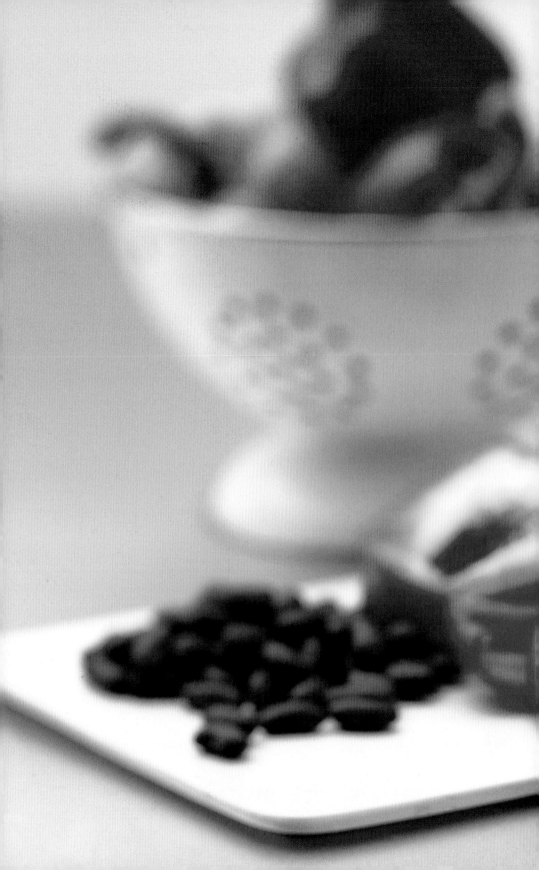

vegetarian

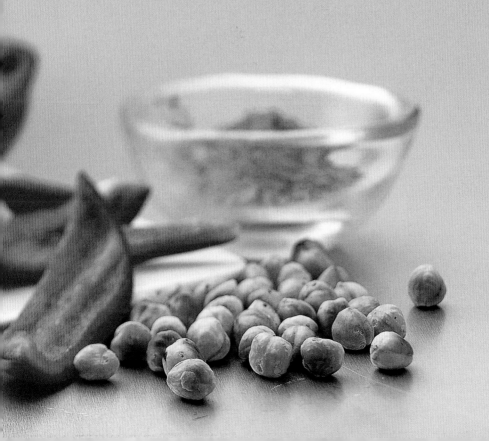

Nutritional values

Kcals 345 (1435 Kj)

fat 8 g

protein 11 g

carbohydrate 55 g

Good source of carotene

Preparation time

20 minutes

Cooking time

35 minutes

Serves

4

NUTRITIONAL TIP

This meal provides the ideal balance of starchy foods – count each serving as 2–3 portions when checking your daily intake. Camargue red rice is particularly high in fibre.

red rice and pumpkin risotto

Grown in the Camargue region of France, red rice is a wholegrain wild rice with a nutty flavour that complements the delicate flavour of pumpkin and makes a quick-to-prepare fork supper full of rustic French flavour.

1 litre (1¾ pints) vegetable stock

250 g (8 oz) Camargue red rice

1 tablespoon olive oil

1 onion, finely chopped

2 garlic cloves, finely chopped

750 g (1½ lb) pumpkin, peeled, deseeded and diced

5 tablespoons fresh basil or oregano, finely chopped, plus extra leaves to garnish

50 g (2 oz) fresh Parmesan, coarsely grated

salt and pepper

Parmesan shavings, to garnish

1 Bring the stock to the boil in a saucepan then add the rice and simmer for 35 minutes.

2 Meanwhile, heat the oil in a frying pan, add the onion and cook for 5 minutes, stirring occasionally until softened. Add the garlic, pumpkin and a little salt and pepper, mix together then cover and cook over a moderate heat for 10 minutes, stirring occasionally until softened.

3 Drain the rice and reserve the cooking liquid. Stir the chopped herbs into the frying pan along with the drained rice and grated Parmesan. Adjust the seasoning and moisten with the reserved rice liquid if needed.

4 Spoon into shallow dishes and garnish with extra herbs and Parmesan shavings.

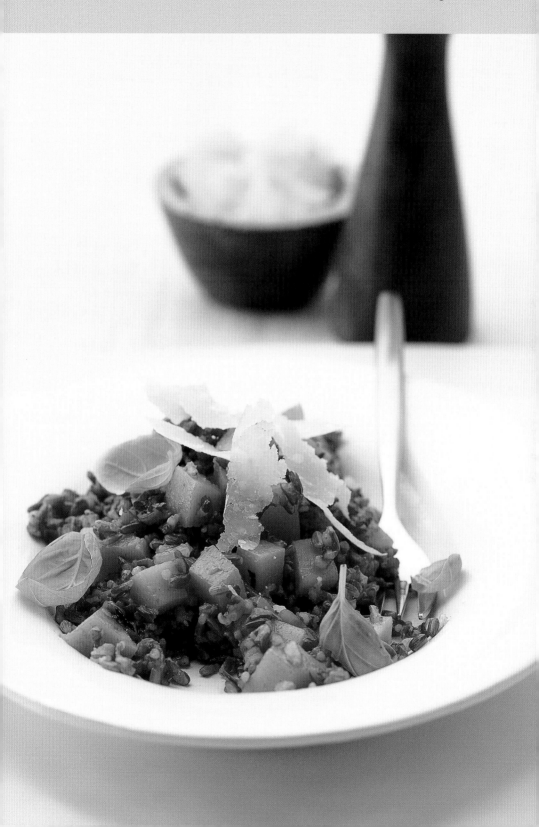

Nutritional values

Kcals 225 (945 Kj)

fat 10 g

protein 14 g

carbohydrate 21 g

Good source of fibre

Preparation time

25 minutes

Cooking time

1 hour 25 minutes

Serves

4

 NUTRITIONAL TIP

Not only are soya beans an excellent source of protein and fibre, but they also contain phytoestrogens. The butternut squash boosts levels of carotenoids.

butternut squash
and soya bean curry

This light, mild-tasting curry has a gingery kick that complements the flavour of the butternut squash. Serve with warmed naan bread, cucumber raita and hot pickles for those who like a bit of extra heat.

1 tablespoon sunflower oil

1 onion, chopped

2 garlic cloves, finely chopped

1 teaspoon fennel seeds, lightly crushed

2 cm (¾ inch) fresh root ginger, peeled and finely chopped

1 tablespoon mild curry paste

400 g (13 oz) can chopped tomatoes

450 ml (¾ pint) vegetable stock

250 g (8 oz) cooked soya beans

400 g (13 oz) butternut squash, peeled, deseeded and diced

small bunch of coriander leaves, to garnish

1 Heat the oil in a saucepan, add the onion and cook for 5 minutes, stirring occasionally until softened. Stir in the garlic, fennel seeds, ginger and curry paste and cook for 1 minute.

2 Mix in the canned tomatoes, stock and beans and bring to the boil, stirring. Cover and simmer for 40 minutes.

3 Stir in the butternut squash, cover again and cook for a further 35 minutes, stirring occasionally until just tender. If there seems to be more liquid than you would like, remove the lid for the last 15 minutes of cooking.

4 Spoon the curry into serving bowls with cooked rice, garnish with the coriander leaves, top with small spoonfuls of cucumber raita, garnish with coriander leaves and serve with warmed naan bread.

Nutritional values

Kcals 365 (1530 Kj)

fat 17 g

protein 17 g

carbohydrate 38 mg

Good source of carotenoids

Preparation time

25 minutes, plus cooling

Cooking time

30–38 minutes

Serves

4

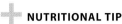 **NUTRITIONAL TIP**

Spinach provides the carotenoid lutein. Serve the polpettes with a glass of fresh orange juice so that the vitamin C in the orange juice can aid the absorption of the iron in the spinach during digestion.

spinach and feta polpettes

These Greek-inspired potato cakes are made with frozen spinach for ease and flavoured with crumbled feta cheese and nutmeg, then lightly fried in olive oil and served with a fresh tomato and garlic sauce.

500 g (1 lb) old potatoes, cut into chunks

375 g (12 oz) frozen spinach, defrosted and well drained

200 g (7 oz) feta cheese, drained and coarsely grated

¼ teaspoon ground nutmeg

50 g (2 oz) wholemeal plain flour

2 tablespoons sunflower or olive oil

salt and pepper

TOMATO SAUCE
1 tablespoon olive oil

1 onion, finely chopped

2 garlic cloves, finely chopped

500 g (1 lb) tomatoes, skinned and diced

2 teaspoons sun-dried or ordinary tomato purée

1 Bring a large saucepan of water to the boil, add the potatoes and simmer for 18–20 minutes until just tender.

2 Drain the potatoes, tip them back into the dry pan and mash. Stir in the drained spinach, feta, nutmeg and salt and pepper and mix well.

3 Spoon the mixture into 12 mounds on a chopping board then leave until cool enough to shape.

4 Meanwhile, make the tomato sauce by heating the oil in a saucepan, add the onion and garlic and cook for 5 minutes until softened and lightly browned. Stir in the tomatoes, tomato purée and a little salt and pepper and simmer for 5 minutes until pulpy.

5 Pat the spinach mixture into rounds with floured hands then coat lightly in the flour. Heat 1 tablespoon of the oil in a frying pan then add the spinach rounds, cooking them in batches and adding remaining oil as needed. Fry for 2–3 minutes each side until golden, then drain on kitchen paper.

6 Arrange the polpettes on serving plates with spoonfuls of tomato sauce.

Nutritional values
Kcals 385 (1610 Kj)
fat 26 g
protein 9 g
carbohydrate 29 g
Good source of vitamin E

Preparation time
25 minutes
Cooking time
30–35 minutes
Serves
4

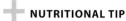 **NUTRITIONAL TIP**
Nuts and a wholegrain topping make this into a high-fibre dish. Although it is fairly high in fat, this is mainly monounsaturated and therefore a good choice.

mushroom and hazelnut streusel

Richly flavoured with balsamic vinegar and garlic, this delicious mushroom stew is topped with a crumbly hazelnut, oat and sage streusel then baked until golden. Serve with steamed carrots and stir-fried cabbage for a completely balanced meal.

STREUSEL TOPPING
50 g (2 oz) wholemeal flour

50 g (2 oz) oats

50 g (2 oz) soya margarine

50 g (2 oz) hazelnuts, chopped

3 tablespoons chopped sage, plus extra leaves to garnish

BASE
2 tablespoons olive oil

1 onion, chopped

3 flat mushrooms, sliced

375 g (12 oz) mixed cup and shitaake mushrooms, halved

2 garlic cloves, finely chopped

2 tablespoons wholemeal flour

300 ml (½ pint) vegetable stock

2 tablespoons balsamic vinegar

1 tablespoon tomato purée

1 teaspoon Dijon mustard

salt and pepper

1 To make the topping, put the flour, oats and margarine in a bowl and rub the fat into the flour with your fingertips until the mixture resembles fine breadcrumbs. Stir in the hazelnuts and sage and set aside.

2 Heat 1 tablespoon of the oil in a large frying pan, add the onion and cook for 5 minutes, stirring occasionally until they are softened.

3 Add the remaining oil then mix in the mushrooms and garlic. Cook for 3–4 minutes, stirring until lightly browned.

4 Sprinkle the flour over the mushrooms then mix in. Pour the stock into the pan, add the vinegar, tomato purée, mustard and salt and pepper and bring to the boil, continuing to stir gently.

5 Transfer the mushroom mixture to a shallow 1.8 litre (3 pint) ovenproof dish. Sprinkle the streusel mixture over the top and bake in a preheated oven, 190°C (375°F, Gas Mark 5), for 20–25 minutes until the topping is browned. Garnish with extra sage leaves and serve.

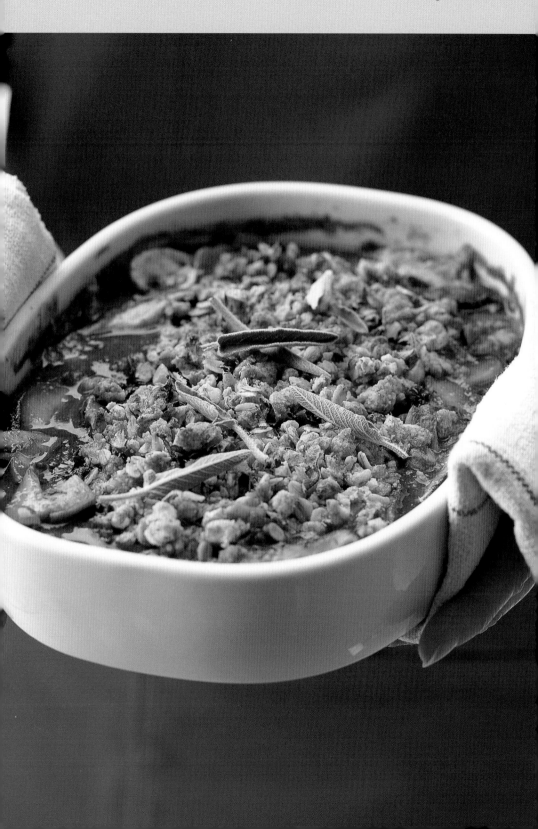

Nutritional values

Kcals 335 (1415 Kj)

fat 14 g

protein 13 g

carbohydrate 43 g

Good source of fibre

Preparation time

30 minutes

Cooking time

1 hour 40 minutes

Serves

4–5

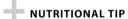 **NUTRITIONAL TIP**

This brightly coloured, high-fibre bake is packed with carotenoids, folate, potassium, iron and calcium.

beetroot and red bean bake

This wonderfully mellow dish is flavoured with Spanish smoked paprika (known as pimentón), cumin seeds and cinnamon. Served with a colourful chunky salsa and brown rice, it is an ideal supper to share with friends.

1 tablespoon sunflower oil

1 onion, chopped

2 garlic cloves, finely chopped

2 carrots, diced

625 g (1¼ lb) raw beetroot, peeled and diced

1 teaspoon ground pimentón

½ teaspoon ground cinnamon

1 teaspoon cumin seeds, roughly crushed

410 g (13¼ oz) can red kidney beans, drained

400 g (13 oz) can chopped tomatoes

600 ml (1 pint) vegetable stock

salt and pepper

fromage frais, to serve

chopped coriander, to garnish

1 Heat the oil in a frying pan, add the onion and cook for 5 minutes, stirring occasionally until softened.

2 Stir in the garlic, carrots and beetroot then mix in the ground spices and cumin seeds. Cook for 1 minute then mix in the kidney beans, tomatoes and stock and season with salt and pepper. Bring to the boil, stirring, then transfer to an ovenproof casserole dish.

3 Cover and transfer to a preheated oven, 180°C (350°F, Gas Mark 4). Cook for 1½ hours.

4 Spoon the stew on to plates, top with spoonfuls of a salsa of avocado, red onion and tomato and fromage frais and garnish with chopped coriander leaves.

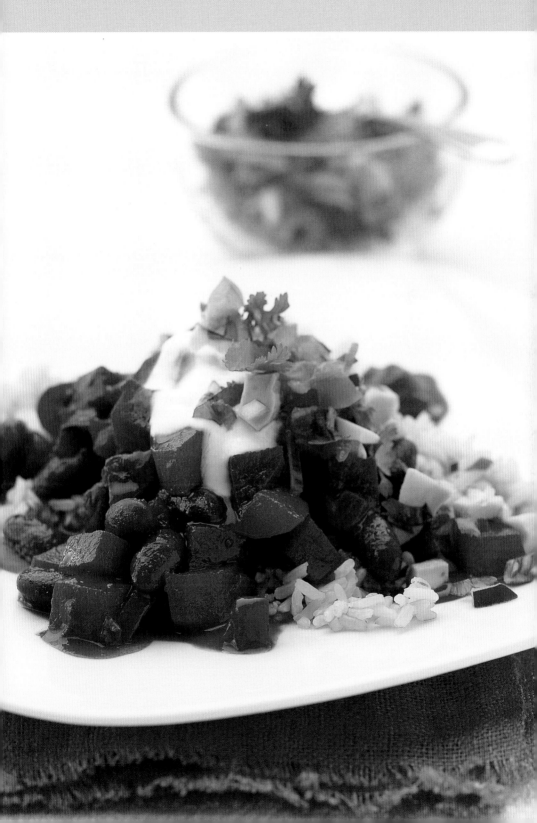

Nutritional values

Kcals 480 (2015 Kj)

fat 14 g

protein 25 g

carbohydrate 68 g

Good source of fibre

Preparation time

30 minutes

Cooking time

35 minutes

Serves

4

NUTRITIONAL TIP

A high-fibre supper dish that will boost your vegetable intake, this is a good source of carotenoids, folate and calcium with additional protective substances (isothiacyanates) from the cabbage.

cheesy lentil and vegetable pie

Comfort food at its best, this tasty carrot and baked bean base is full of fibre. It is topped with a cheesy bubble and squeak mixture, and then baked in the oven until golden.

1 tablespoon sunflower oil

1 onion, finely chopped

500 g (1 lb) carrots, diced

2 garlic cloves, finely chopped

415 g (13½ oz) can low-sugar, low-salt baked beans

125 g (4 oz) red lentils

450 ml (¾ pint) vegetable stock

salt and pepper

TOPPING
750 g (1½ lb) baking potatoes

150 g (5 oz) Savoy cabbage, finely shredded

3–4 tablespoons semi-skimmed milk

100 g (3½ oz) Cheddar cheese, grated

1 Heat the oil in a saucepan, add the onion and cook for 5 minutes, stirring occasionally until softened.

2 Stir in the carrots and garlic and cook for 2 minutes. Mix in the baked beans, lentils and stock, salt and pepper. Bring to the boil, cover and simmer for 20 minutes until the lentils are tender, adding extra liquid if needed.

3 Meanwhile, make the topping. Cut the potatoes into large chunks and cook in the base of a steamer half-filled with boiling water for 15 minutes. Add the steamer top, fill with the cabbage, cover and cook for 5 minutes until both cabbage and potatoes are tender.

4 Drain the potatoes, return to the pan and mash with the milk. Stir in the cabbage, two-thirds of the cheese and season with salt and pepper.

5 Spoon the hot carrot mixture into the base of a 1.5 litre (2½ pint) pie dish. Spoon the potato mixture on top then sprinkle with the remaining cheese. Grill for 5 minutes until golden-brown. Serve with frozen peas.

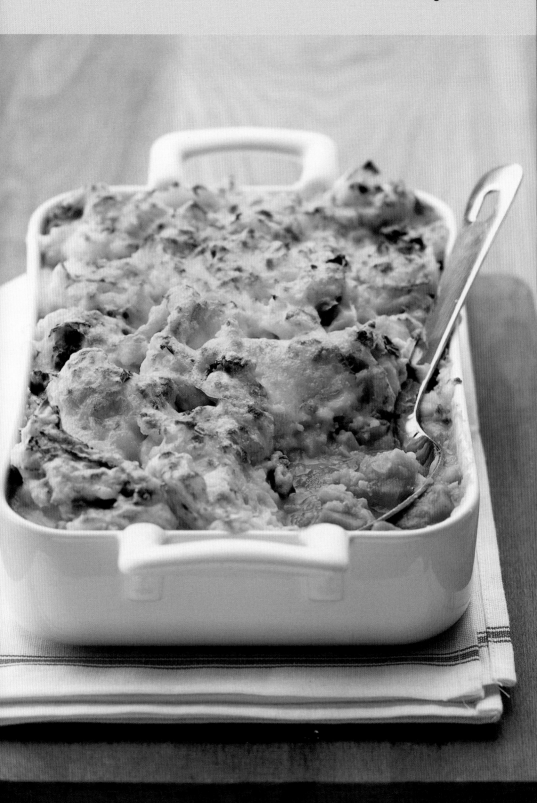

Nutritional values

Kcals 427 (1380 Kj)

fat 20 g

protein 14 g

carbohydrate 50 g

Good source of beta-carotene

Preparation time

15 minutes

Cooking time

16–17 minutes

Serves

4

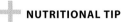 **NUTRITIONAL TIP**

Eat plenty of green leafy vegetables as they are rich in carotenoids, folate and iron. The wholegrain noodles boost the fibre content.

Thai coconut greens with soba

Quick and easy to prepare, this creamy smooth curry is flavoured with Thai red curry paste for a gentle heat then finished with tangy fresh coriander leaves and a sprinkling of crunchy dry-roasted peanuts, and served on a bed of noodles.

1 tablespoon sunflower oil

1 onion, chopped

4 teaspoons Thai red curry paste

400 ml (14 fl oz) can reduced-fat coconut milk

150 ml (¼ pint) vegetable stock

1 carrot, cut into matchsticks

100 g (3½ oz) purple sprouting broccoli

125 g (4 oz) pak choi

small bunch of fresh coriander

100 g (3½ oz) green beans, thickly sliced

200 g (7 oz) soba (wholewheat Japanese noodles)

75 g (3 oz) frozen peas (optional)

50 g (2 oz) dry-roasted unsalted peanuts

1 Heat the oil in a saucepan, add the onion and cook for 5 minutes, stirring occasionally until softened. Stir in the curry paste and cook for 1 minute.

2 Stir in the coconut milk and stock, then add the carrot sticks. Cover and simmer for 5 minutes.

3 Meanwhile, thickly slice the broccoli stems and halve the florets. Cut the leaves from the pak choi and shred. Cut the white stems into matchstick strips. Reserve some coriander for a garnish, then roughly chop the rest.

4 Add the green beans and broccoli stems to the pan, cover again and cook for 3 minutes. Half-fill a second saucepan with water, bring to the boil then add the soba. Simmer for 3–5 minutes until just cooked, then drain.

5 Add the broccoli florets, pak choi strips and leaves and peas (if using) to the curry and cook for 2 minutes.

6 Spoon the soba into mounds in 4 shallow dishes. Stir the chopped coriander into the curry then spoon the vegetables on top of the soba and the sauce into the base of the dish. Garnish with the peanuts and the reserved coriander.

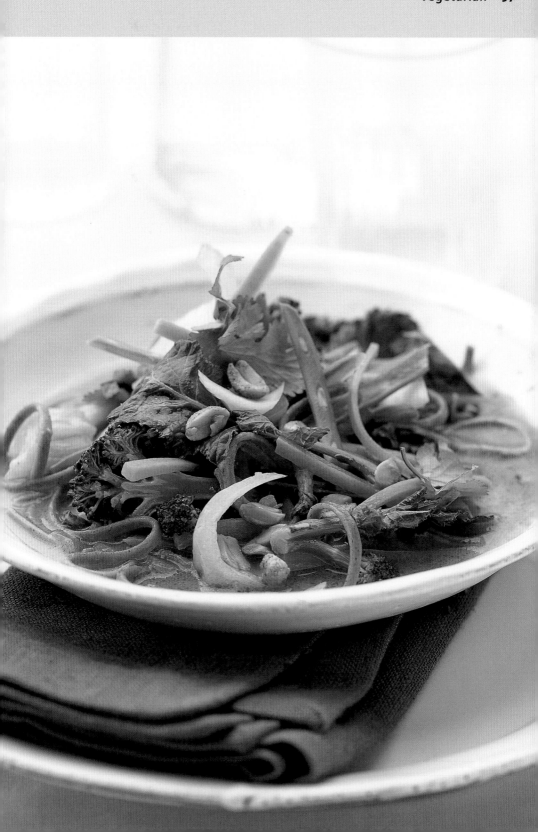

Nutritional values

Kcals 525 (2190 Kj)

fat 32 g

protein 11 g

carbohydrate 52 g

Good source of fibre

Preparation time

35 minutes, plus chilling

Cooking time

20 minutes

Serves

4

NUTRITIONAL TIP

Red and orange peppers are good sources of vitamin C, beta-carotene and bioflavonoids. Garlic and onions have sulphur-containing compounds that may protect against stomach cancer.

ratatouille and oatmeal tarts

These colourful tarts are made with a dairy-free, nutty-tasting wholemeal and oatmeal flour pastry case flavoured with chopped rosemary and filled with a garlicky mix of rosemary-flavoured Mediterranean vegetables.

PASTRY

175 g (6 oz) wholemeal plain flour

50 g (2 oz) medium oatmeal

4 teaspoons finely chopped fresh rosemary

125 g (4 oz) soya margarine

2–3 tablespoons water

salt and pepper

FILLING

1 tablespoon olive oil

1 onion, chopped

2 garlic cloves, finely chopped

1 red and 1 orange pepper, cored, deseeded and diced

375 g (12 oz) courgettes, diced

400 g (13 oz) can chopped tomatoes

2 teaspoons sugar

1 tablespoon finely chopped fresh rosemary, plus extra leaves to garnish

1 To make the pastry, put the flour and oatmeal in a bowl with the chopped rosemary and salt and pepper. Add the margarine and rub in until the mixture resembles fine breadcrumbs. Stir in enough water to mix to a smooth dough.

2 Knead the pastry lightly then roll out on a lightly floured surface. Use to line 4 individual 12 cm (5 inch) tins. Trim the top edge and prick the base with a fork. Chill for 15 minutes.

3 Line the pastry cases with greaseproof paper then fill with baking beans. Bake in a preheated oven, 190°C (375°F, Gas Mark 5), for 10 minutes, remove the paper and beans and cook for 10 more minutes until the pastry is lightly browned.

4 Meanwhile, make the filling by heating the oil in a frying pan. Add the onion and cook until softened. Stir in the garlic, diced peppers and courgettes and cook for 3 minutes.

5 Stir in the tomatoes, sugar, rosemary and a little salt and pepper. Simmer for 5 minutes until thick.

6 Carefully remove the tart cases from the hot tins, put on a serving plate and fill with the ratatouille mixture. Garnish with extra rosemary and serve with a jacket potato and salad.

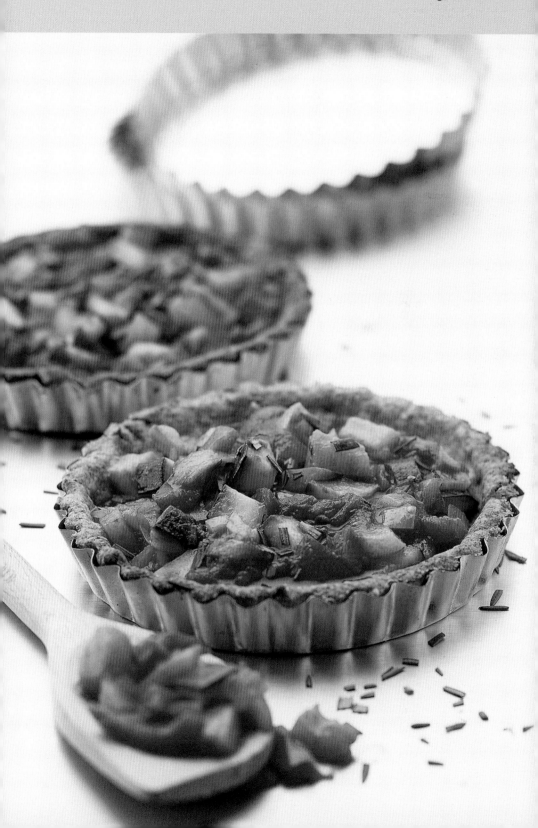

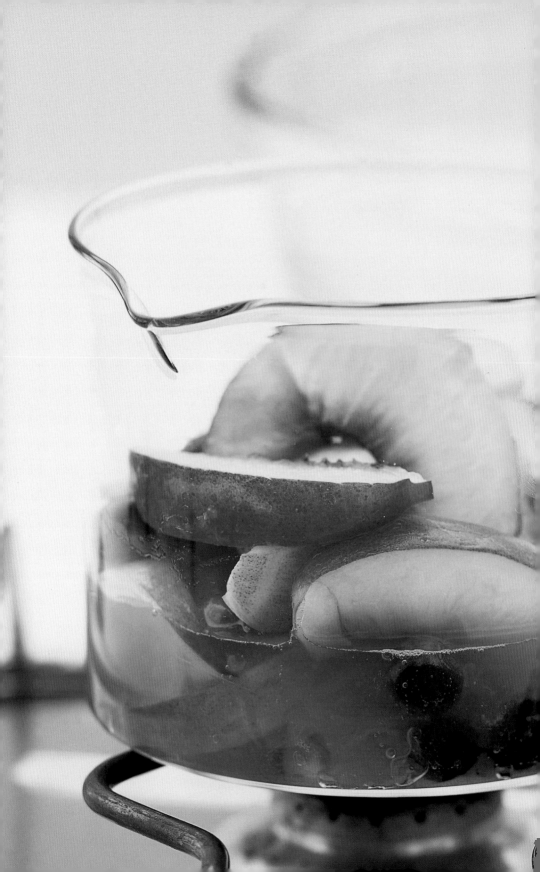

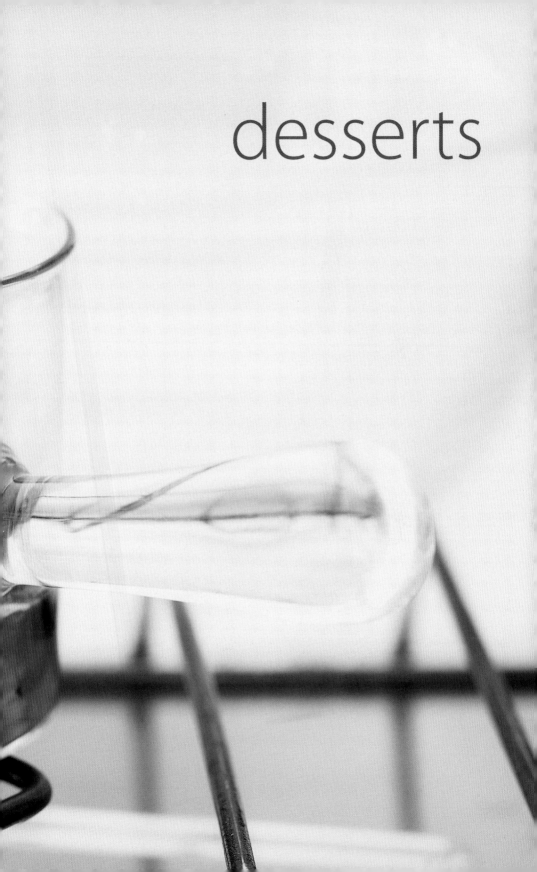

desserts

Nutritional values

Kcals 70 (305 Kj)

fat 0 g

protein 0 g

carbohydrate 19 g

Good source of vitamin C

Preparation time

25 minutes, plus freezing

Cooking time

4–5 minutes

Serves

4

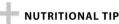 **NUTRITIONAL TIP**

Low in fat but packed with vitamins, mangoes are rich in beta-carotene and vitamin C, both of which are vital antioxidants.

lime and mango granita

Light, tangy and refreshing, this is the perfect dessert to follow a spicy curry or chilli. It's also a good way to encourage those members of the family who are not too keen on fruit to be a little more adventurous.

50 g (2 oz) caster sugar

300 ml (½ pint) water

finely grated rind and juice of 2 limes

1 large ripe mango

lime rind curls, to decorate

mango slices, to serve

1 Put the sugar, water and lime rind into a small saucepan and heat gently for 4–5 minutes until the sugar has completely dissolved. Leave to cool.

2 Cut a thick slice off either side of the mango to reveal the large, flat stone, then make criss-cross cuts in these slices and scoop the flesh away from the skin using a spoon. Cut away the flesh surrounding the stone and remove and discard the skin. Purée the mango flesh in a liquidizer or food processor until smooth.

3 Mix the mango purée, sugar syrup and lime juice together then pour into a shallow roasting tin so that it is about 2 cm (¾ inch) deep. Freeze for 1 hour.

4 Take the tin out of the freezer and mash the mixture with a fork to break up any large ice crystals. Return to the freezer and freeze for 1½ hours, beating with a fork at 30-minute intervals until the granita has the consistency of crushed ice.

5 Spoon into 4 dishes, decorate with the lime rind curls and serve with extra slices of mango. Transfer any remaining granita to a plastic container with a lid and return to the freezer.

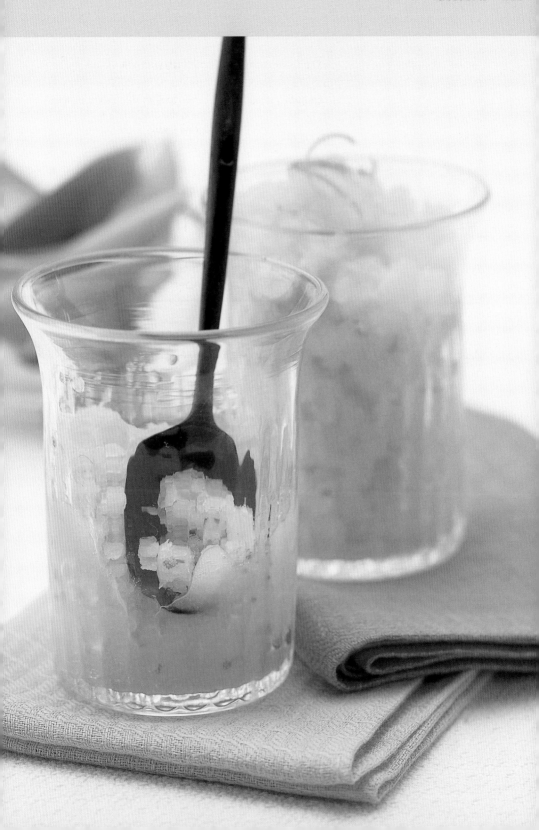

Nutritional values

Kcals 130 (1325 Kj)

fat 3 g

protein 3 g

carbohydrate 43 g

Preparation time

15 minutes

Cooking time

5–7 minutes

Serves

4

NUTRITIONAL TIP

Because the eggs are only lightly cooked, do not serve this to a new mum, young child or anyone convalescing from illness. This dessert is rich in vitamin C, magnesium and iron.

mixed fruit sabayon

Give a simple fruit salad the star treatment by bathing it in a light, bubbly whisked custard sauce cooked over a saucepan of simmering water. Choose ripe fruits to give maximum natural sweetness.

175 g (6 oz) or 4 fresh apricots, halved, stoned and sliced

200 g (7 oz) strawberries, halved or quartered, depending on size

150 g (5 oz) seedless red grapes, halved if large

2 kiwifruit, each peeled and cut into 8 long, thin slices

2 egg yolks

25 g (1 oz) caster sugar

5 tablespoons sparkling white grape and elderflower juice

icing sugar, for dusting

1 Divide the fruit among 4 shallow ovenproof dishes.

2 Half-fill a saucepan with water, bring to the boil and set a large bowl over the top, checking that the base of the bowl does not touch the water.

3 Add the egg yolks, sugar and juice to the bowl and whisk, using a balloon or electric whisk, for 4–5 minutes until the mixture is very thick and frothy and leaves a trail when the whisk is lifted.

4 Pour the frothy custard over the fruits and place under a preheated grill for 1–2 minutes until just browned. Dust lightly with sifted icing sugar and serve immediately.

Nutritional values

Kcals 315 (1325 Kj)

fat 4 g

protein 11 g

carbohydrate 43 g

Source of beta-carotene

Preparation time

25 minutes, plus rising

Cooking time

20 minutes

Serves

6

 NUTRITIONAL TIP

Plums provide beta-carotene and the carotenoid cryptoxanthin. If the plums are very sweet, reduce the amount of sugar by half. Serving with fromage frais adds extra calcium.

buckwheat blinis with red plum and cinnamon compote

These delicate little yeast pancakes are made with a mixture of buckwheat and white flour and cooked in a similar way to drop scones. Serve them warm, topped with spoonfuls of cinnamon-spiced plums and fromage frais.

250 g (8 oz) buckwheat flour

125 g (4 oz) strong plain white flour

pinch of salt

1 teaspoon fast-action dried yeast

300 ml (½ pint) semi-skimmed milk

150 ml (¼ pint) water, plus extra 3 tablespoons

1 egg, beaten

oil, for greasing

fromage frais, to serve

PLUM COMPOTE
500 g (1 lb) ripe red plums, halved, pitted and sliced

50 g (2 oz) caster sugar

¼ teaspoon ground cinnamon

2 tablespoons water

1 Put the flours, salt and yeast in a bowl and mix together. Heat the milk and water in a small saucepan until warm to touch. Gradually stir into the flour to form a smooth batter.

2 Cover the bowl with a clean tea towel and leave it in a warm place for 1 hour until the batter is well risen and bubbling.

3 Meanwhile, make the compote. Put the plums in a saucepan with the sugar, cinnamon and water. Cover and cook gently for 5 minutes until tender. Set aside until needed.

4 Stir the beaten egg and 3 tablespoons warm water into the batter. Heat a lightly oiled griddle or heavy-based frying pan. Drop spoonfuls of the blini mixture well spaced apart on to the griddle or into the frying pan. Cook for 2–3 minutes until golden on the underside then flip and cook the other side.

6 Wrap the cooked blinis in a tea towel to keep warm. Brush the pan with more oil until all the mixture has been used.

7 Reheat the compote. Divide the blinis among 6 plates, top with the warm compote and spoonfuls of fromage frais, spooning a little of the compote juice over the fromage frais.

Nutritional values

Kcals 385 (1600 Kj)

fat 20 g

protein 15 g

carbohydrate 37 g

Good source of vitamin C

Preparation time

20 minutes, plus freezing

Cooking time

2–2½ hours

Serves

4

✚ **NUTRITIONAL TIP**

Milk is an excellent source of calcium and vitamin D and makes a delicious ice cream. The fruit is a valuable source of antioxidants, beta-carotene and bioflavonoids.

pistachio kulfi with papaya

This popular Indian ice cream is delicately flavoured with cardamom and pistachios. Because it is made by slowly boiling milk until it is reduced to about one-third of its original volume, it is much healthier than European ice creams.

1.5 litres (2½ pints) full-fat milk

3 cardamom pods, roughly crushed

2 tablespoons caster sugar

50 g (2 oz) pistachio nuts, skinned and finely chopped, plus extra to decorate

TO DECORATE
1 papaya

½ pomegranate (optional)

1 Pour the milk into a large heavy-based saucepan and bring to the boil. Add the cardamom pods and their black seeds, reduce the heat and simmer for 2–2½ hours until the milk has reduced to about 450 ml (¾ pint).

2 Strain the milk through a sieve, stir in the caster sugar and leave to cool.

3 Stir the pistachio nuts into the milk then pour the mixture into 4 tall, thin moulds. Freeze overnight until firm.

4 To serve, halve the papaya, scoop out the black seeds then peel. Cut into thin slices and put in a bowl. Break the pomegranate into large pieces and remove the pink seeds. Add these to the bowl, cover and chill until needed.

5 To turn out the kulfi, dip the moulds into just boiled water, count to 10 then quickly invert the moulds on to individual plates. Remove the moulds and clean the plates with kitchen paper if needed. Spoon the fruit around the kulfi and decorate with extra pistachio nuts, cut into thin slivers.

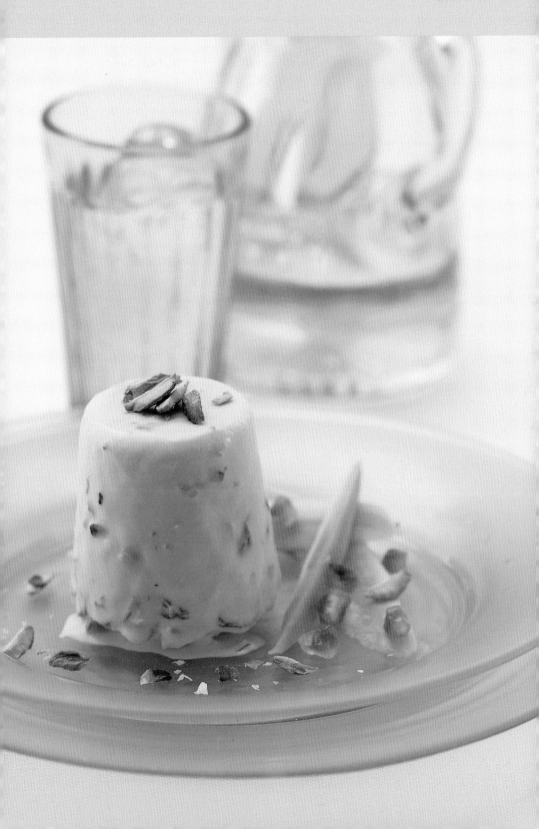

Nutritional values

Kcals 230 (970 Kj)

fat 3 g

protein 6 g

carbohydrate 49 g

Good source of fibre

Preparation time

20 minutes

Cooking time

5 minutes

Serves

4

NUTRITIONAL TIP

Grape juice is 100 per cent pure fruit juice and makes a pleasant change from apple or orange juice. Red or black grapes are a good source of antioxidants and are a delicious addition to this low-fat dessert.

spiced pears with ratafia

This light low-fat dessert is delicately flavoured with mulled wine spices and cooked in naturally sweet red grape juice and topped with spoonfuls of fromage frais mixed with crushed almond-flavoured biscuits.

4 ripe Comice or Williams pears

450 ml (¾ pint) unsweetened red grape juice

1 cinnamon stick, halved

¼ teaspoon ground nutmeg

pared rind of 1 orange

2 tablespoons light muscovado sugar

4 teaspoons cornflour

50 g (2 oz) ratafia biscuits, crumbled

200 g (7 oz) low-fat fromage frais

1 Peel the pears, leaving the stalks on, then halve them, cutting down through the stalks. Scoop out the cores with a teaspoon.

2 Put the pears in a saucepan with the grape juice, spices, orange rind and sugar. Heat gently for 5 minutes until tender. Set aside so that the flavours can develop.

3 Lift the pears out of the pan and reserve. Discard the orange peel. Mix the cornflour in a bowl with a little water to form a smooth paste. Pour into the spiced grape juice then bring to the boil, stirring until thickened and smooth. Add the pears and warm through.

4 Stir the biscuit crumbs into the fromage frais. Spoon the pears into 4 dishes and add spoonfuls of the fromage frais mixture.

Nutritional values

Kcals 280 (1185 Kj)

fat 7 g

protein 11 g

carbohydrate 45 g

Good source of calcium

Preparation time

25 minutes

Cooking time

40 minutes

Serves

4

 NUTRITIONAL TIP

A traditional dessert is adapted here to include berries and lemon rind, containing the protective compounds flavanoids and terpenoid.

queen of puddings

This delicious old English dessert is wonderfully indulgent, yet low in fat. Traditionally made with a layer of berry jam, here a small amount of jam is mixed with fresh blueberries to reduce the calories and boost the vitamin content.

450 ml (¾ pint) semi-skimmed milk

50 g (2 oz) fresh breadcrumbs

grated rind of 2 lemons

100 g (3½ oz) caster sugar

3 eggs, separated

2 tablespoons red cherry or strawberry jam

100 g (3½ oz) blueberries

1 Pour the milk into a saucepan and bring just to the boil. Remove from the heat and stir in the breadcrumbs, lemon rind and 2 tablespoons of the caster sugar.

2 Leave the mixture to cool for a few minutes then gradually beat in the egg yolks, one at a time. Pour the mixture into a 1.2 litre (2 pint) ovenproof pie dish and leave to stand for 10 minutes.

3 Bake the lemon custard in a preheated oven, 180°C (350°F, Gas Mark 4), for 20–25 minutes until set and just beginning to brown.

4 Reduce the oven temperature to 160°C (325°F, Gas Mark 3). Whisk the egg whites in a large bowl to form stiff, moist-looking peaks. Gradually whisk in the remaining sugar a dessertspoonful at a time. When all the sugar has been added, whisk for 1–2 minutes until the meringue is thick and glossy.

5 Dot the lemon custard with the jam and sprinkle with the blueberries. Spoon the meringue over the blueberries and swirl with a spoon. Return the dish to the oven and cook for 15 minutes until the meringue is a pale biscuit colour. Serve warm or cold.

Nutritional values

Kcals 95 (405 Kj)

fat 0 g

protein 2 g

carbohydrate 23 g

Preparation time

15 minutes, plus chilling

Cooking time

4–5 minutes

Serves

6

NUTRITIONAL TIP

Frozen fruits have just the same nutritional value as fresh ones and are a much cheaper option when fresh ones are out of season. The red berries here are packed with flavonoids.

red berry terrine

Convenience foods are not all bad. Here a pack of frozen berry fruits has been mixed with a carton of pure unsweetened red grape juice and set with a little gelatine to make an easy fresh fruity dessert, which is high in vitamins and low in calories.

450 ml (¾ pint) unsweetened red grape juice

2 x 12 g (½ oz) sachets powdered gelatine

50 g (2 oz) caster sugar

500 g (1 lb) bag frozen mixed berry fruits

few extra defrosted or fresh fruits, to decorate (optional)

1 Measure 150 ml (¼ pint) of the grape juice into a bowl, sprinkle over the gelatine, making sure that all the powder has been absorbed by the juice. Set aside for 5 minutes.

2 Stand the bowl in a saucepan of simmering water and heat gently for 4–5 minutes until the gelatine has completely dissolved.

3 Stir the sugar into the gelatine mixture then mix with the remaining grape juice.

4 Pour the still-frozen fruits into a 1 kg (2 lb) loaf tin then cover with the warm juice mixture. Mix together then chill in the fridge for 3 hours until set and the fruits have defrosted fully.

5 To serve, dip the loaf tin into a bowl of just-boiled water. Count to 10, then loosen the edge of the jelly and turn out on to a serving plate. If liked, decorate with a few extra fruits and serve the jelly cut into thick slices.

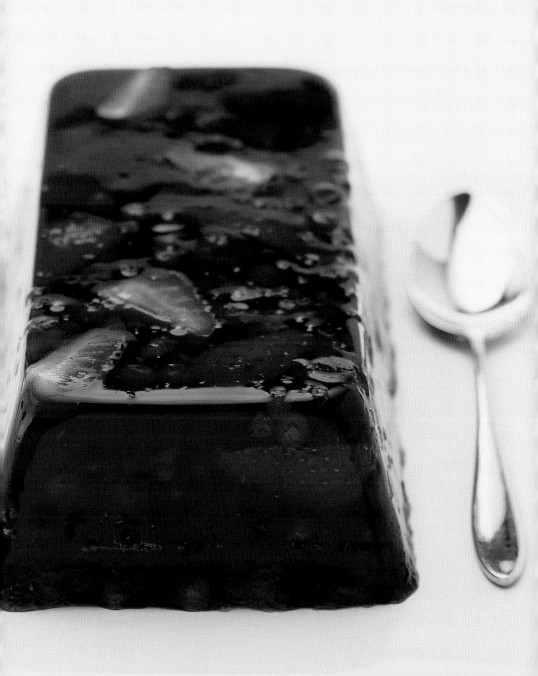

Nutritional values

Kcals 75 (310 Kj)

fat 4 g

protein 1 g

carbohydrate 9 g

Preparation time

15 minutes

Cooking time

6–8 minutes

Serves

12

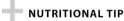 **NUTRITIONAL TIP**

Two tarts count as a portion of fruit, with the berries providing valuable flavonoids. Boost your calcium intake by serving with fromage frais or yogurt ice cream.

mini nectarine and blueberry tarts

These little tarts are made with wafer-thin pieces of filo pastry brushed lightly with melted butter and oil and baked until golden. Even with the addition of melted butter these tarts are much lower in fat than ones made with shortcrust pastry.

25 g (1 oz) butter, melted

2 teaspoons olive oil

4 sheets of filo pastry, defrosted if frozen, each 30 x 18 cm (12 x 7 inches), or 65 g (2½ oz) total weight

2 tablespoons low-sugar red berry jam

juice of ½ orange

4 ripe nectarines, halved, stoned and sliced

150 g (5 oz) blueberries

icing sugar, for dusting

fromage frais or yogurt ice cream, to serve

1 Heat the butter and oil in a small saucepan until the butter has melted.

2 Unroll the pastry and separate into sheets. Brush lightly with the butter mixture, then cut into 24 pieces, each 10 x 8 cm (4 x 3½ inches).

3 Arrange a piece in each of the sections of a deep 12-hole muffin tin then add a second piece at a slight angle to the first pieces to give a pretty jagged edge to each pastry case.

4 Bake in a preheated oven, 180°C (350°F, Gas Mark 4), for 6–8 minutes until golden. Meanwhile, warm the jam and orange juice in a saucepan then add the nectarines and blueberries and warm through.

5 Carefully lift the tart cases out of the muffin tin and transfer to a serving dish. Fill with the warm fruits and dust with sifted icing sugar. Serve with spoonfuls of fromage frais or yogurt ice cream.

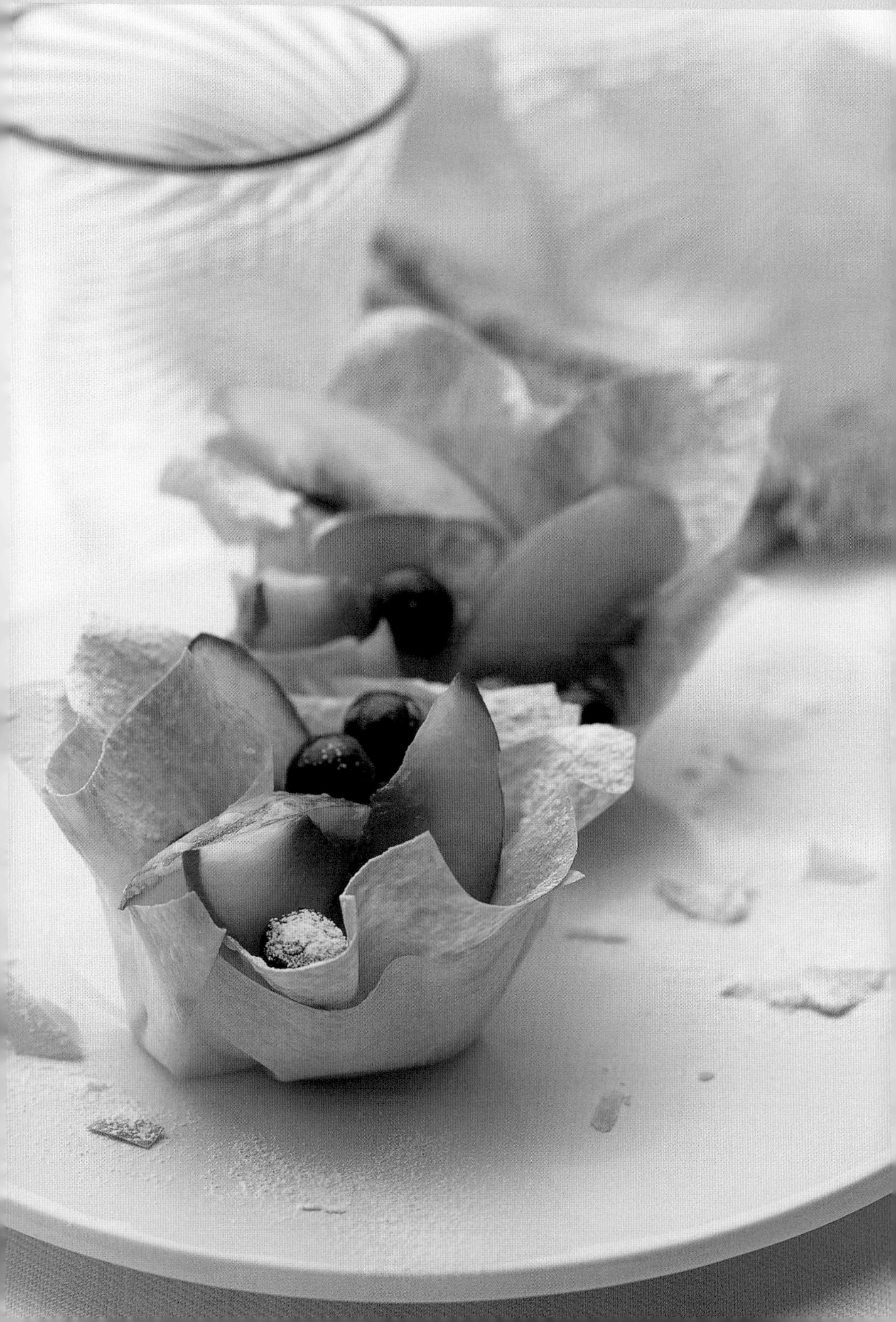

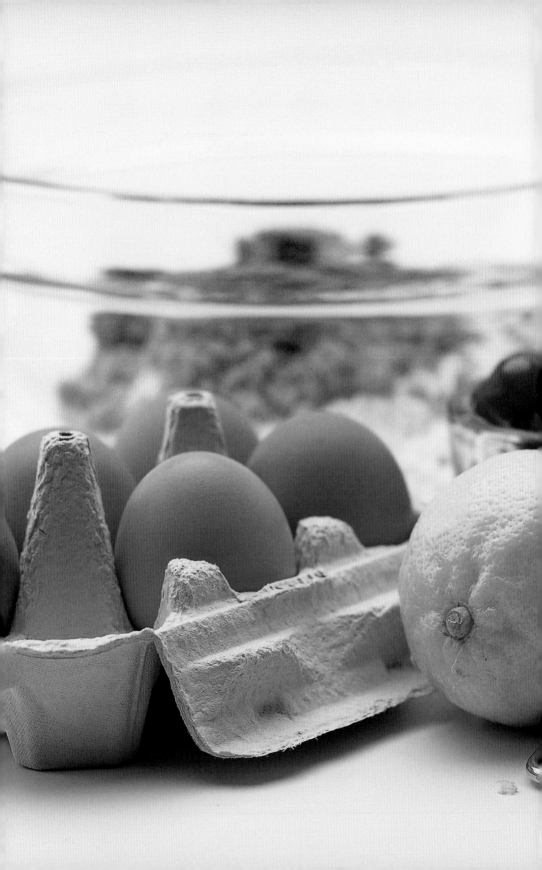

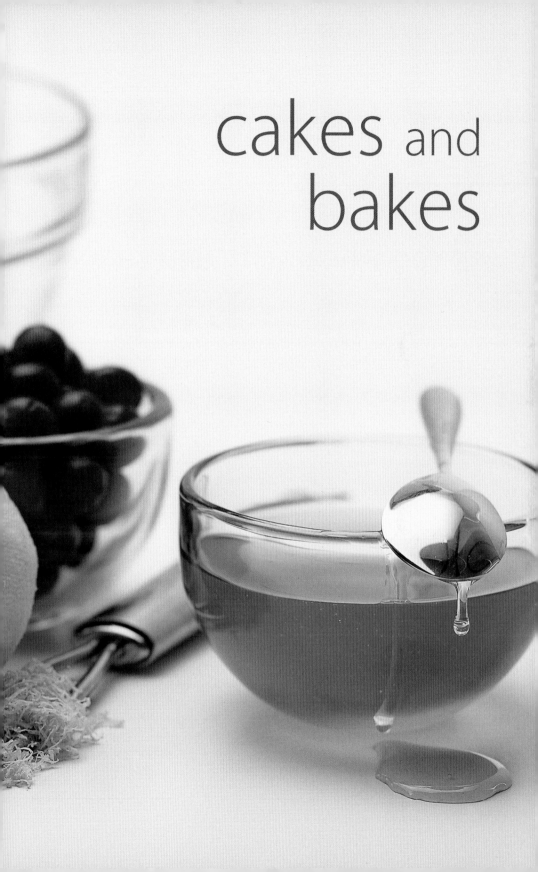

cakes and
bakes

Nutritional values

Kcals 185 (780 Kj)

fat 11 g

protein 5 g

carbohydrate 20 g

Good source of vitamin E

Preparation time

30 minutes

Cooking time

25–30 minutes

Makes

18

✚ NUTRITIONAL TIP

The mix of wholemeal flour, wheatgerm and fruit goes to make up a cake that is rich in beta-carotene, vitamin E and other carotenoids. One slice counts as one starch portion for the day.

spiced wheatgerm and carrot cake

You would never guess that this light, moist cake is made with reduced fat and sugar. Delicately spiced with cinnamon and glacé ginger, these moreish pieces are topped with cream cheese and extra spice.

200 g (7 oz) carrots, grated

1 dessert apple, grated

grated rind of ½ orange

2 tablespoons glacé ginger

150 ml (¼ pint) sunflower oil

3 eggs, beaten

3 tablespoons wheatgerm

125 g (4 oz) muscovado sugar

200 g (7 oz) self-raising wholemeal flour

2 teaspoons baking powder

1 teaspoon ground cinnamon

FROSTING
200 g (7 oz) low-fat cream cheese

1 tablespoon thick honey

2 tablespoons orange juice

ground cinnamon, to decorate

1 Line a small 18 x 28 x 5 cm (7 x 11 x 2 inch) roasting tin with a large piece of nonstick baking paper, snipping into the corners so that it fits the base and sides of the tin snugly.

2 Put the carrots, apple and orange rind in a bowl and mix in the ginger, oil and eggs.

3 Add all the dry ingredients and mix well. Spoon into the prepared tin, level the surface and bake in a preheated oven, 180°C (350°F, Gas Mark 4), for 25–30 minutes until well risen and the top springs back when pressed with a fingertip.

4 Leave the cake to cool in the tin then turn out and remove the lining paper.

5 Beat together the cream cheese and honey. Gradually mix in the orange juice to form a soft spreadable frosting. Spoon over the cake, swirl with the back of the spoon and sprinkle with a little ground cinnamon. Cut into 18 pieces to serve. Store any leftover cake in the fridge, covered with foil. Use within 2 days.

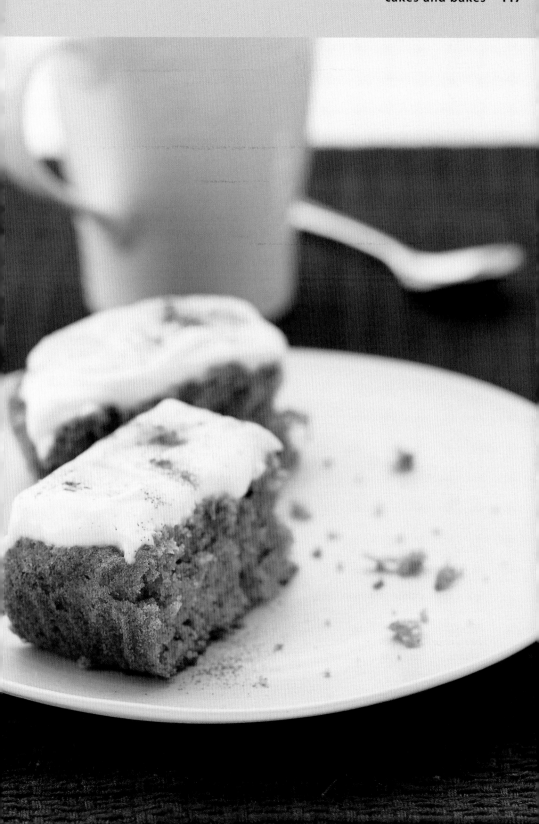

Nutritional values

Kcals 240 (1160 Kj)

fat 5 g

protein 6 g

carbohydrate 46 g

Good source of fibre

Preparation time

25 minutes, plus soaking

Cooking time

1¼ hours

Makes

12–14 slices

 NUTRITIONAL TIP

Packed with fibre, this is a good way to get the family to eat more fibre without them realizing it. It is also a good source of minerals, including calcium and iron.

mixed fruit cake with bran

This looks and tastes just like a traditional fruit cake, but it is packed with fibre and is low in fat. Because it keeps so well in a tin, this cake is ideal to slice and add to lunchboxes or to satisfy the mid-morning munchies.

175 g (6 oz) high-fibre wheat bran breakfast cereal

375 g (12 oz) luxury mixed dried fruit

450 ml (¾ pint) apple or grape juice

150 g (5 oz) soft light muscovado sugar

175 g (6 oz) self-raising flour

2 teaspoons baking powder

1 teaspoon ground cinnamon

½ teaspoon ground nutmeg

grated rind and juice of 1 orange

2 eggs, beaten

50 g (2 oz) halved pecan nuts

1 Put the cereal and dried fruit in a bowl, pour the apple or grape juice over the top and leave to soak for 30 minutes.

2 Line the base and sides of a 20 cm (8 inch) round springform tin with nonstick baking paper.

3 Mix the dry ingredients together in a bowl. Stir the orange rind and juice into the soaked cereal then combine the mixture with the dry ingredients and eggs.

4 Spoon into the prepared tin, level the surface and arrange the nuts over the top.

5 Bake in a preheated oven, 160°C (325°F, Gas Mark 3), for 1 hour 10 minutes to 1¼ hours, or until well risen and a skewer inserted into the centre of the cake comes out cleanly. Check the cake after 20 minutes and cover with foil if the nuts appear to be browning too quickly.

6 Leave the cake to cool, then remove from the tin, peel away the lining paper and serve, cut into slices. Store the cake in an airtight tin for up to a week.

Nutritional values

Kcals 150 (640 Kj)

fat 8 g

protein 8 g

carbohydrate 14 g

Contains beta-carotene

Preparation time

35 minutes

Cooking time

15–20 minutes

Makes

8 slices

 NUTRITIONAL TIP

Cutting down on saturated fats can be hard, especially if you love baking. However, the fat in this cake comes predominately from ground almonds and is monounsaturated.

baked almond and apricot slice

This fluffy almond sponge filled with a fruity apricot purée and creamy fromage frais makes the perfect centrepiece to any teatime. Unlike a traditional Victoria sponge, this is made without butter and flavoured with ground almonds so is much lower in fat.

4 eggs

125 g (4 oz) caster sugar

½ teaspoon almond essence

50 g (2 oz) plain flour

75 g (3 oz) ground almonds

2 tablespoons flaked almonds

sifted icing sugar, to decorate

APRICOT FILLING
125 g (4 oz) ready-to-eat dried apricots

150–200 ml (5–7 fl oz) water or apple juice

125 g (4 oz) low-fat fromage frais

1 Put the eggs, caster sugar and almond essence in a large bowl and whisk until very thick and frothy.

2 Sift the flour into the bowl then gently fold the flour and ground almonds into the egg mixture.

3 Divide the mixture between 2 18 cm (7 inch) round baking tins, greased and lined with greaseproof paper. Tilt the tins to level the surface of the mixture rather than using a knife, then sprinkle flaked almonds over one of the cakes.

4 Bake in a preheated oven, 180°C (350°F, Gas Mark 4), for 15–20 minutes until the cakes are risen, golden-brown and the top springs back when pressed lightly with a fingertip. Cool for 10 minutes, then loosen the edges with a knife and turn out on to a wire rack to cool. Peel off the lining papers.

5 Put the apricots in a small saucepan with the water or apple juice. Cover and simmer for 10 minutes until softened. Purée in a blender or food processor until smooth. Leave to cool.

6 Put the cake without the flaked almonds on a serving plate, spread over the apricot purée then top with fromage frais. Add the second cake, almond side uppermost, and dust lightly with sifted icing sugar. Cut into slices to serve.

Nutritional values

Kcals 275 (1160 Kj)

fat 10 g

protein 7 g

carbohydrate 42 g

Moderate source of fibre

Preparation time

25 minutes

Cooking time

1–1¼ hours

Makes

10 slices

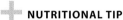 **NUTRITIONAL TIP**

Cranberries are rich in potassium, beta-carotene and vitamin C and contain natural antioxidants, such as quercetin.

cranberry, honey and banana loaf

This easy fork-together, 'cut-and-come again' cake stores well. Serve it sliced as a healthy snack or add it to packed lunchboxes. Dried cranberries have been used here, but you may like to experiment with the addition of different dried fruits.

50 g (2 oz) vegetable margarine or butter

125 g (4 oz) soft light muscovado sugar

3 tablespoons sunflower oil

3 eggs

500 g (1 lb) bananas, weighed with skins on (about 4)

250 g (8 oz) self-raising wholemeal flour

75 g (3 oz) barley flakes

75 g (3 oz) dried cranberries

1 Line a 1 kg (2 lb) loaf tin with a large piece of nonstick baking paper and snip into the corners so that it fits the base and sides of the tin snugly.

2 Melt the margarine or butter and pour it into a large bowl. Add the sugar, oil and eggs and fork together.

3 Mash the bananas on a plate then add to the sugar mixture with the flour and all but 2 tablespoons of the barley flakes. Mix together, then stir in the dried cranberries.

4 Spoon the mixture into the prepared tin, level the surface and sprinkle with the reserved barley flakes. Cook in a preheated oven, 180°C (350°F, Gas Mark 4), for 1–1¼ hours until well risen and the top has cracked or until a skewer inserted into the centre comes out cleanly. Check after 30 minutes and cover with foil if the top appears to be browning too quickly.

5 Leave the cake to cool in the tin then loosen, turn out and peel off the lining paper. Cut into thick slices to serve. Store in an airtight tin for up to 4 days.

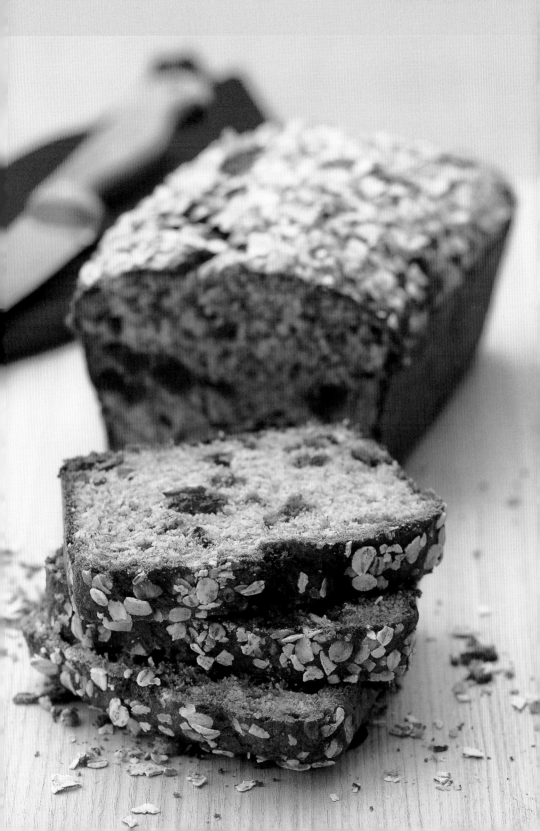

Nutritional values

Kcals 220 (935 Kj)

fat 10 g

protein 5 g

carbohydrate 31 g

Preparation time

15 minutes

Cooking time

18–20 minutes

Makes

12

✚ **NUTRITIONAL TIP**

Each muffin contains potentially protective compounds – bioflavonoids from the blueberries and terpenoid from the grated lemon rind.

blueberry and lemon muffins

Made in minutes, these light fruity muffins are best served while still warm from the oven. They will freeze well in a plastic bag or box. Defrost at room temperature, then warm in the oven or use a microwave.

175 g (6 oz) malthouse or granary flour

125 g (4 oz) plain flour

3 teaspoons baking powder

125 g (4 oz) light muscovado sugar

200 g (7 oz) blueberries

grated rind and juice of 1 lemon

4 tablespoons olive or sunflower oil

50 g (2 oz) vegetable margarine or butter, melted

3 eggs, beaten

150 ml (¼ pint) semi-skimmed milk

LEMON FROSTING (OPTIONAL)
125 g (4 oz) icing sugar, sifted

juice of ½ lemon

1 Put the flours, baking powder, sugar and blueberries in a bowl and mix together. Put the remaining ingredients in a jug and fork together. Add to the dry ingredients and mix briefly with a fork.

2 Divide the mixture among paper cake cases arranged in the sections of a deep 12-hole muffin tin. Cook in a preheated oven, 190°C (375°F, Gas Mark 5), for 18–20 minutes until well risen and the tops are cracked. Leave to cool for 15 minutes in the tin.

3 To make the frosting, sift the icing sugar into a bowl and gradually mix in enough lemon juice to make a thin, spoonable icing. Take the muffins out of the tin and drizzle icing from a spoon in random lines over the top. Leave to harden slightly and serve the muffins while still warm.

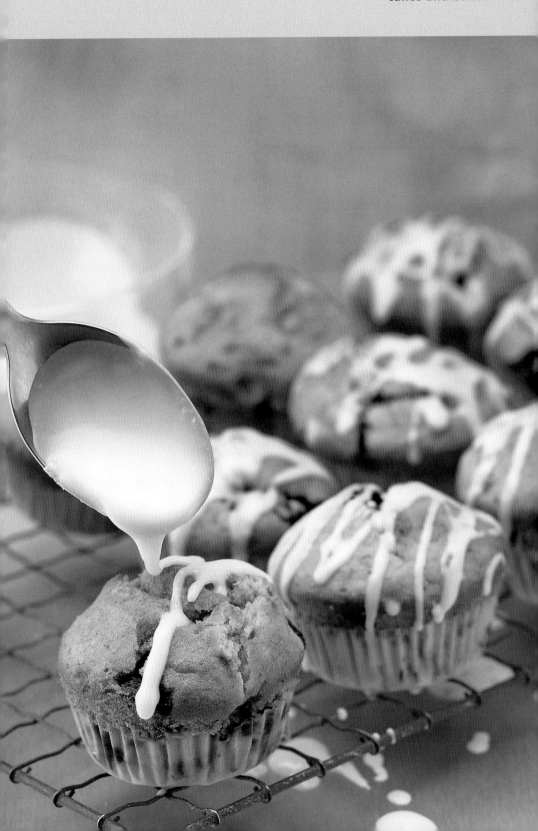

index

references

This book is drawn from a solid scientific foundation and has its basis firmly in research. The following references have provided information for the text:

Food, Nutrition and the Prevention of Cancer: A Global Perspective
World Cancer Research Fund in association with American Institute for Cancer Research, Washington, 1997

Nutritional Aspects of the Development of Cancer
Report of the working group on diet and cancer of the Committee on Medical Aspects of Food and Nutrition Policy. Report on health and social subjects 48.
Department of Health (UK), London, 1998

Diet, Nutrition and the Prevention of Chronic Disease
WHO Technical Report Series 916. Report of joint WHO/FAO Expert Consultation, Geneva, 2003

The Soil Association
www.soilassociation.org

acknowledgements

Executive Editor: Nicola Hill
Project Editor: Kate Tuckett
Executive Art Editor: Rozelle Bentheim
Designer: Beverly Price, one2six creative
Picture Research: Jennifer Veall

picture credits

Special Photography: ©Octopus Publishing Group/William Lingwood

Other Photography: Octopus Publishing Group Limited/Frank Adam 22/ Jean Cazals 25 bottom right/Stephen Conroy 17 centre/Sandra Lane 23 top Getty Images 27 bottom right, 28 bottom left, 29 bottom right

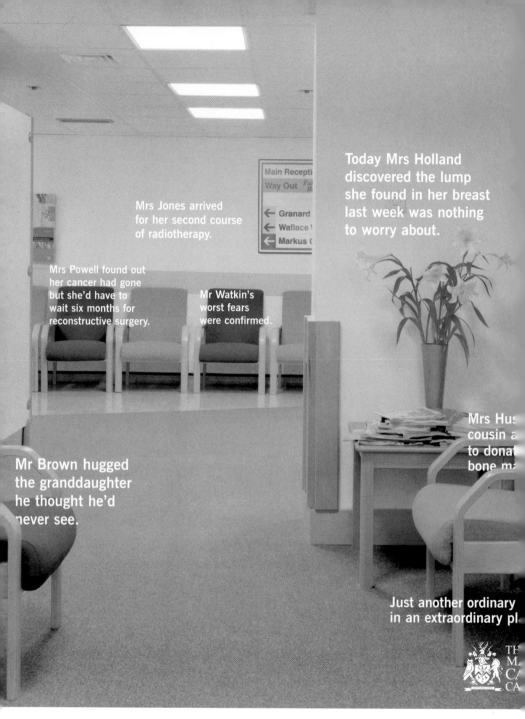

Today Mrs Holland
discovered the lump
she found in her breast
last week was nothing
to worry about.

Mrs Jones arrived
for her second course
of radiotherapy.

Mrs Powell found out
her cancer had gone
but she'd have to
wait six months for
reconstructive surgery.

Mr Watkin's
worst fears
were confirmed.

Mr Brown hugged
the granddaughter
he thought he'd
never see.

Mrs Hus
cousin a
to dona
bone m

Just another ordinary
in an extraordinary pl

Make our day. Donate today.
Please call +44 (0) 20 7808 2233 or visit
www.royalmarsden.org/campaign